Sedentary Behaviour - A Contemporary View

Edited by Adilson Marques and Élvio Rúbio Gouveia

Published in London, United Kingdom

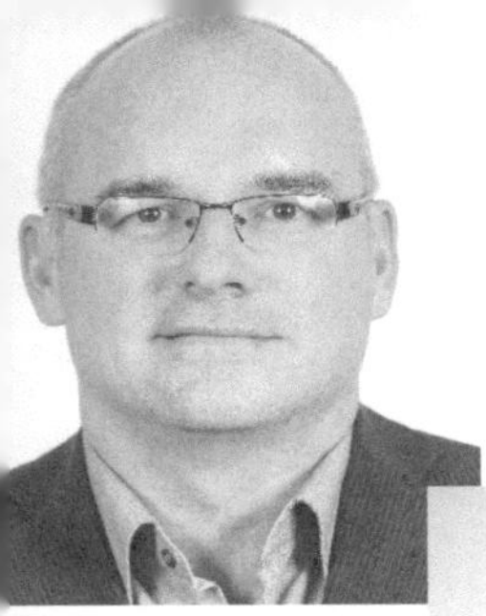
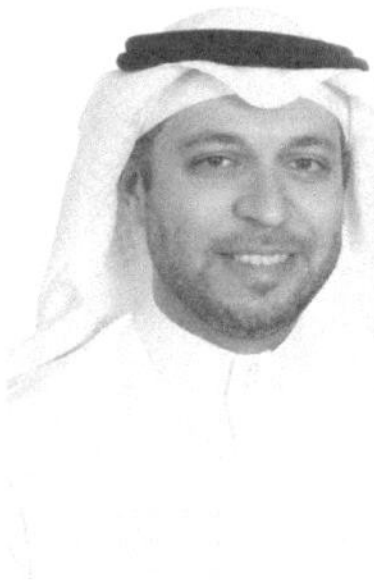
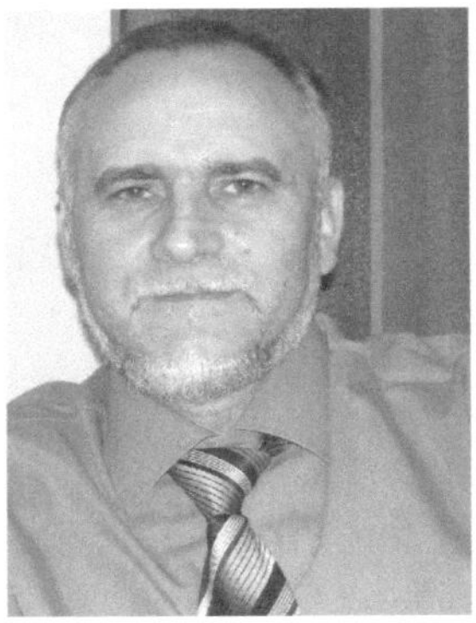
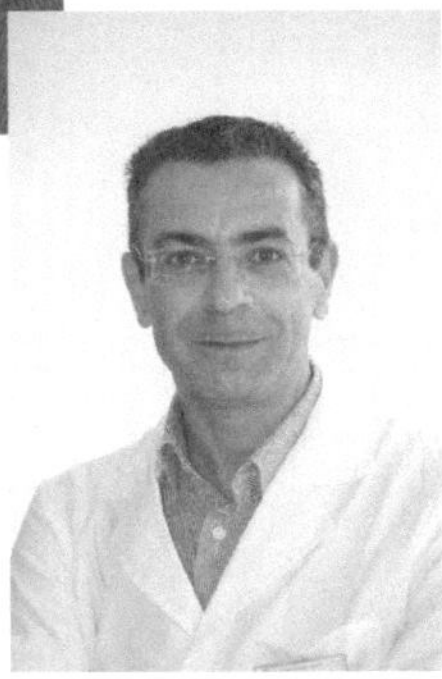
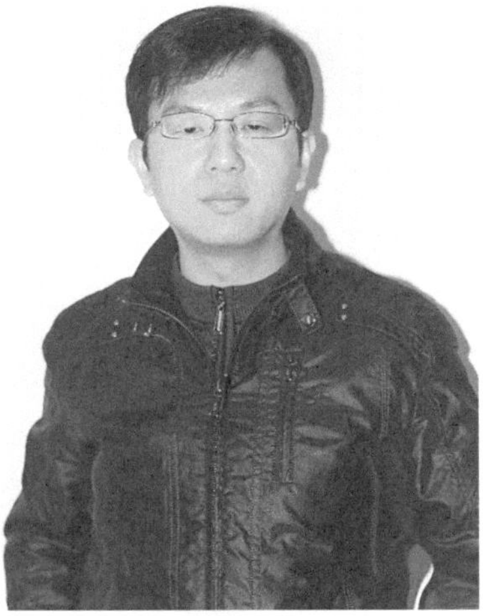
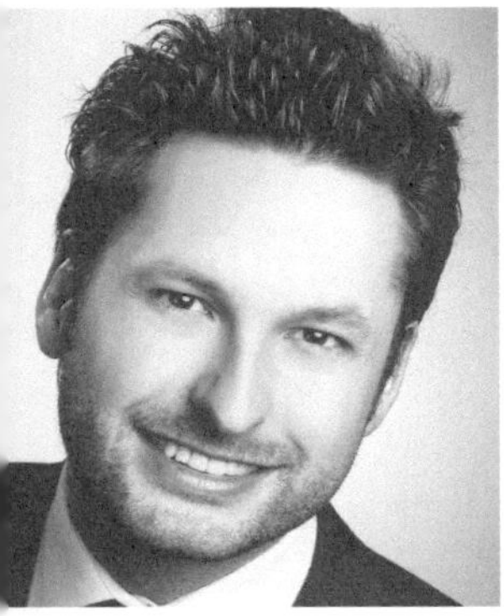
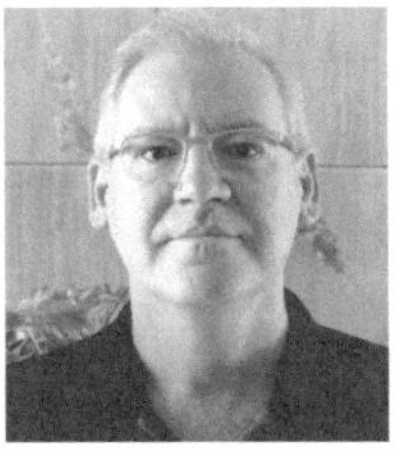

IntechOpen

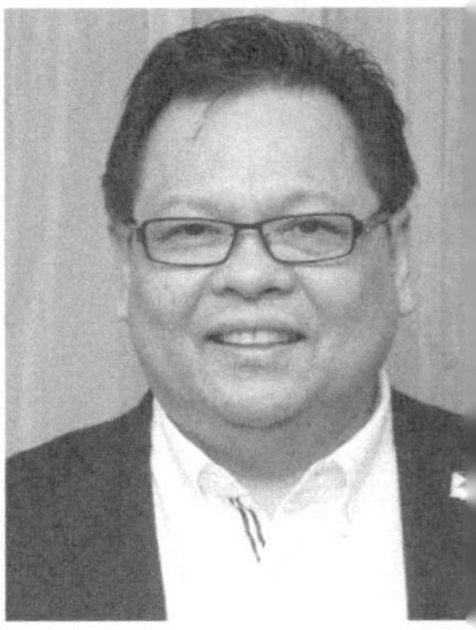
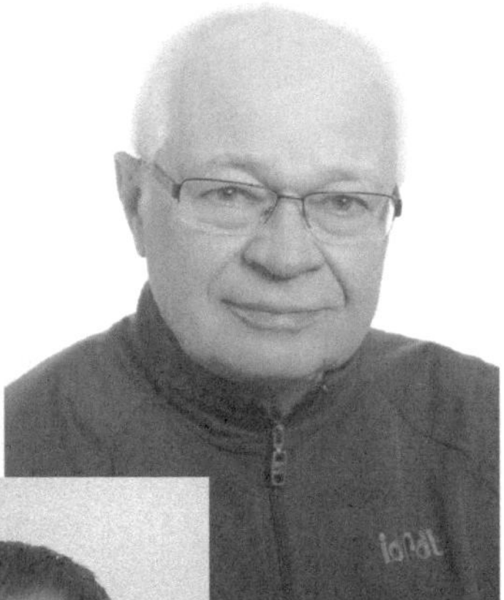
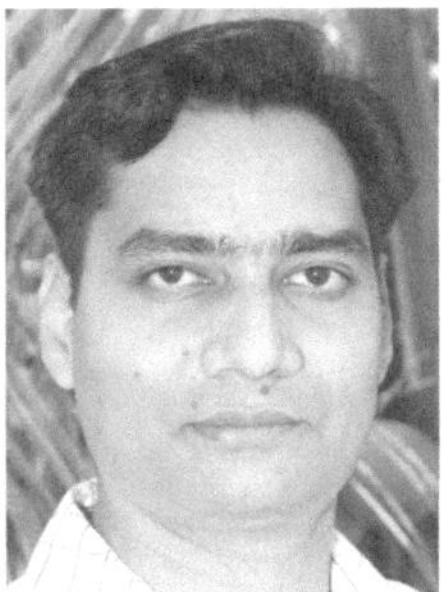
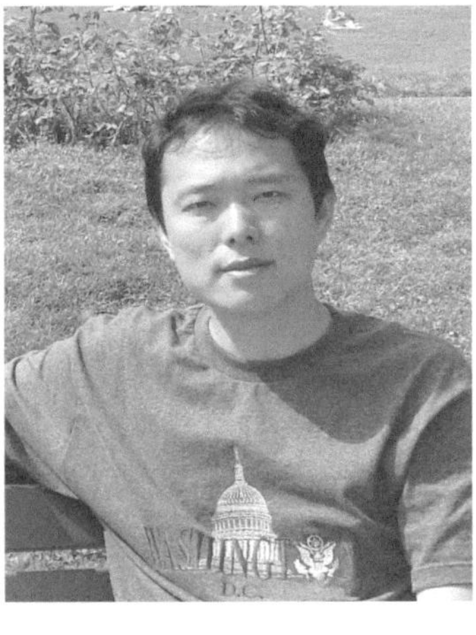
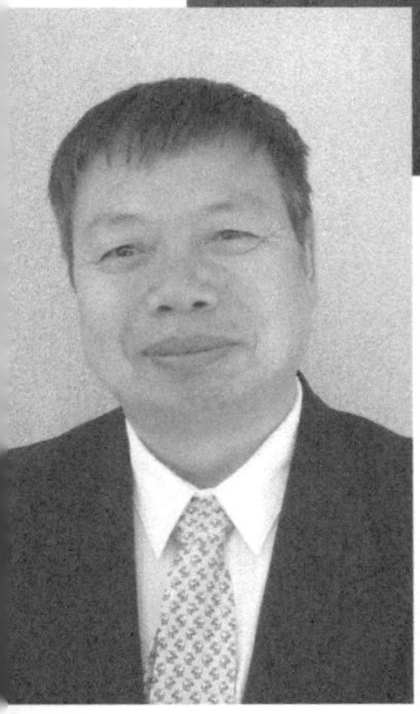
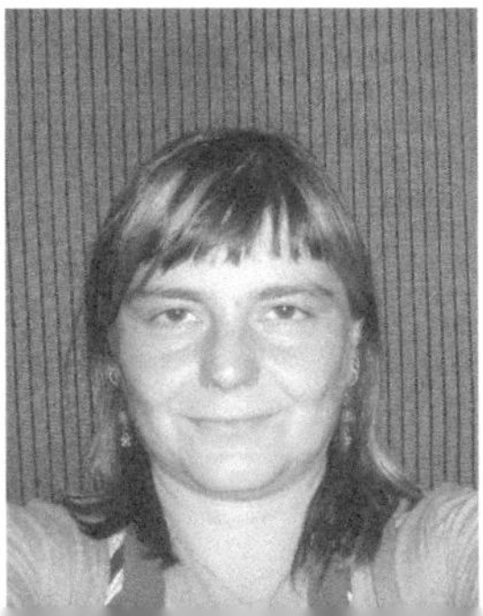

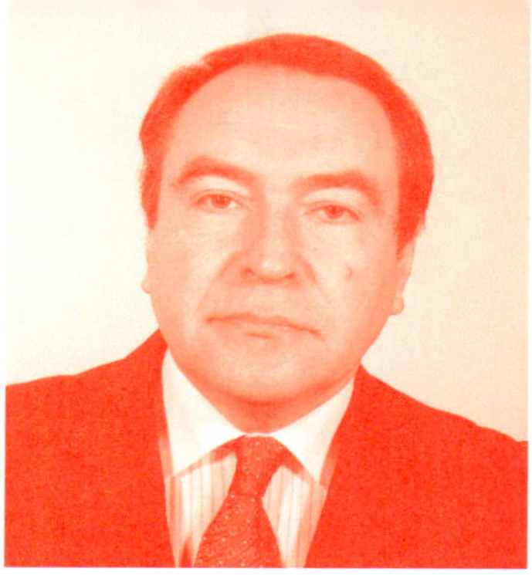
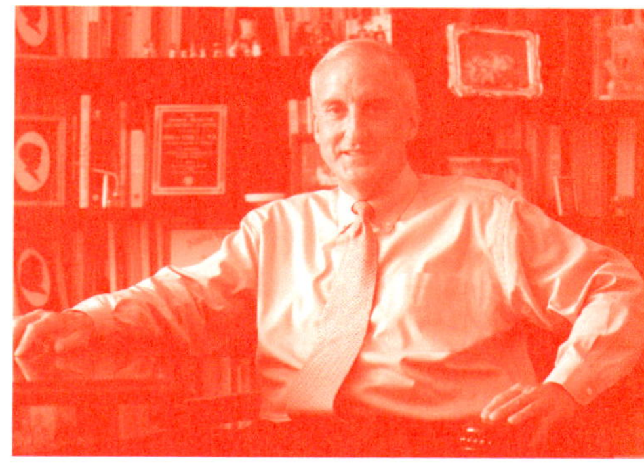
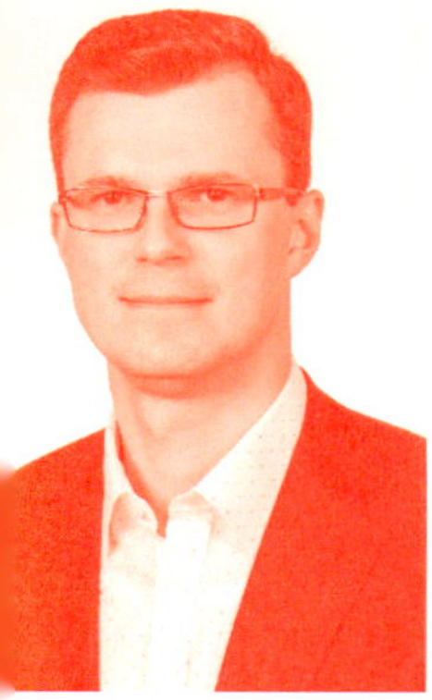
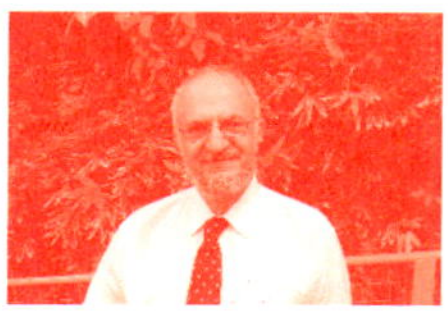
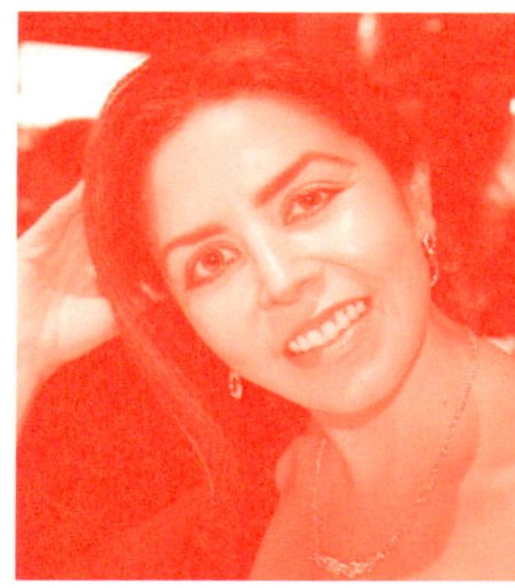

Supporting open minds since 2005

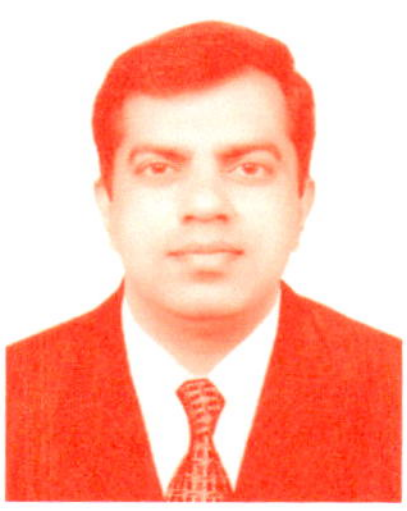
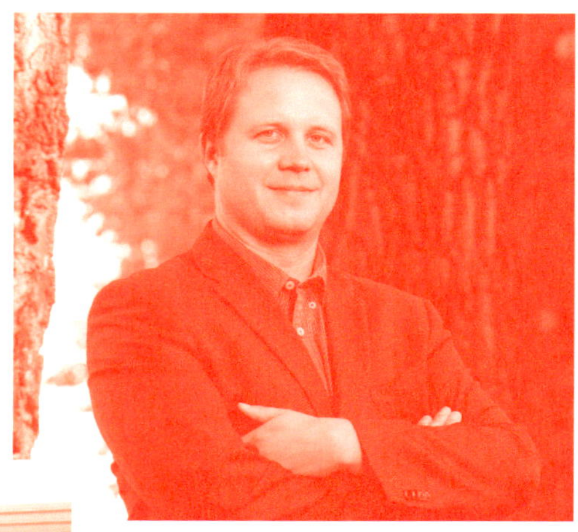
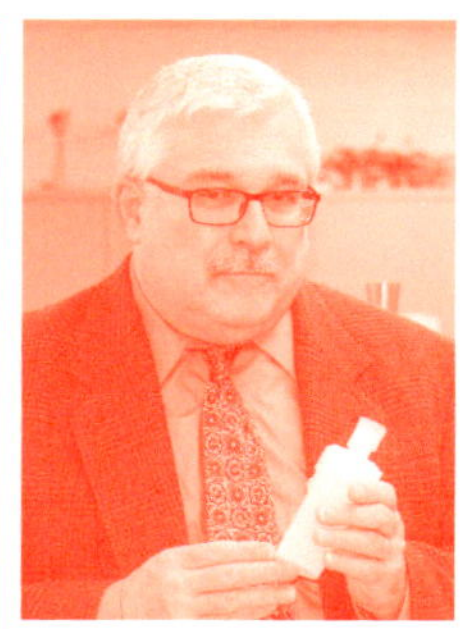
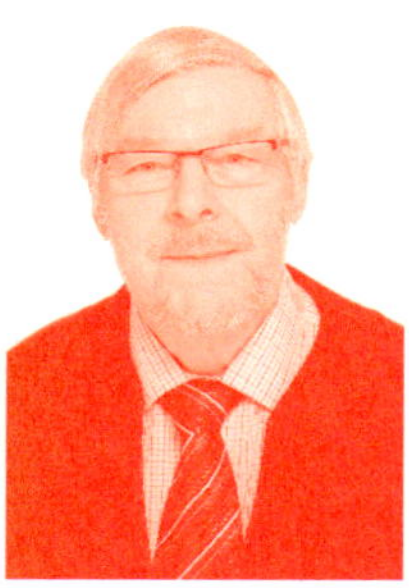
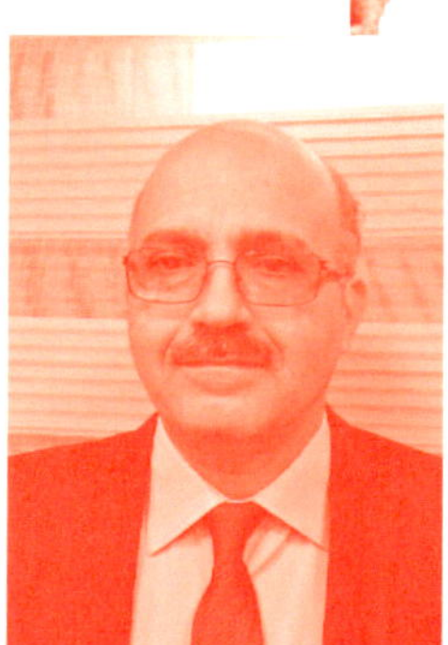
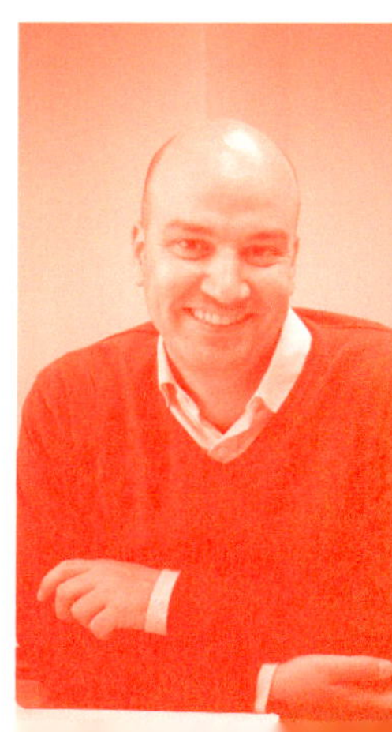
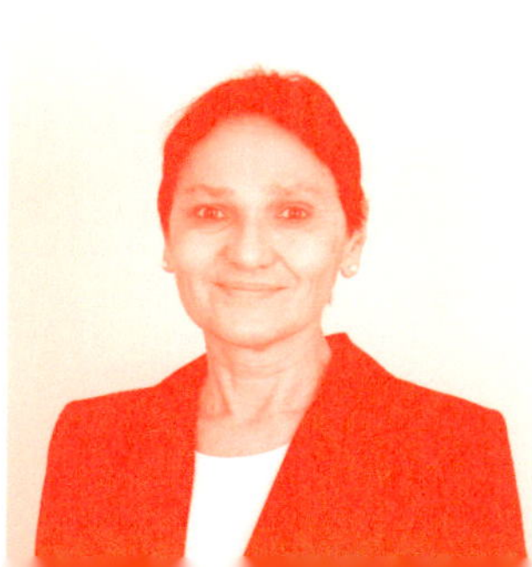

Sedentary Behaviour - A Contemporary View
http://dx.doi.org/10.5772/intechopen.91074
Edited by Adilson Marques and Élvio Rúbio Gouveia

Contributors
Bochen Jia, Olga López Torres, Gabriela F. De Roia, Pablo Lobo, Valeria Baigún, Imtiyaz Ali Mir, Lucy-Joy Wachira, Adilson Marques, Priscila Marconcin, Vera Zymbal, Élvio R. Gouveia, Bruce Jones, Pedro B. Júdice, Gerson Ferrari, André Werneck

First published in London, United Kingdom, 2021 by IntechOpen
IntechOpen is the global imprint of INTECHOPEN LIMITED, registered in England and Wales, registration number: 11086078, 5 Princes Gate Court, London, SW7 2QJ, United Kingdom
Printed in Croatia

British Library Cataloguing-in-Publication Data
A catalogue record for this book is available from the British Library

Additional hard and PDF copies can be obtained from orders@intechopen.com

Sedentary Behaviour - A Contemporary View
Edited by Adilson Marques and Élvio Rúbio Gouveia
p. cm.
Print ISBN 978-1-83968-575-0
Online ISBN 978-1-83968-576-7
eBook (PDF) ISBN 978-1-83968-577-4

Meet the editors

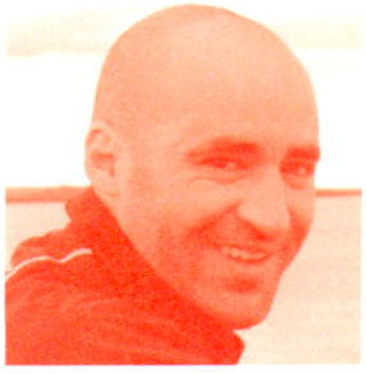

Adilson Marques is an assistant professor at the University of Lisbon, Portugal. He holds bachelor's and master's degrees in Physical Education, a master's in Public Health, a Ph.D. in Sciences of Education, a Ph.D. in Sports Science, and a Ph.D. in Health Sciences. Dr. Marques was a physical education teacher for nine years. His main research interests are health promotion, correlates of physical activity, fitness, sedentary behaviour, and physical education. He has published several international peer-reviewed articles and has been an investigator in several research projects. He is a reviewer for several scientific journals in the field of sports science and health promotion. He is a member of the National Physical Activity Promotion Program at the Portuguese Ministry of Health.

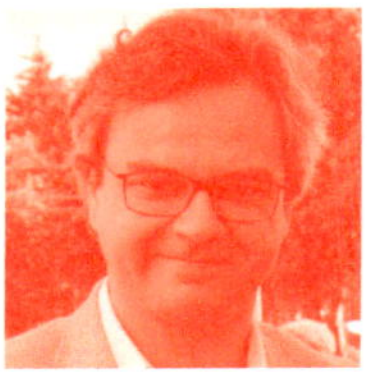

Élvio Rúbio Gouveia has a degree in Physical Education, a master's in Physical Education, and a Ph.D. in Sport Sciences. Currently, Dr. Gouveia is an assistant professor at the University of Madeira, Portugal, and vice president of the Interactive Technologies Institute, a research unit from the Laboratory of Robotics and Engineering Systems. He also collaborates with the Center for the Interdisciplinary Study of Gerontology and Vulnerability, University of Geneva, Switzerland. He has been working on developing and evaluating strategies to promote physical activity, fitness, and quality of life. With a focus on the physiological assessment of human fitness and the promotion of healthy ageing, his research is grounded on a multidisciplinary approach to several issues that affect healthy fitness.

Contents

Preface

Movement behaviours, such as physical activity and sedentary behaviour, are an important public health topic. Physical activity is the most well-known of those behaviours, and its health benefits are unequivocal [1]. However, there is a growing interest in the research of sedentary behaviour around the world.

The interest in studying sedentary behaviour derives primarily from its association to several health outcomes, independent of physical activity, including cardiovascular and metabolic diseases (diabetes, hypertension, dyslipidemia, obesity) [2], cancer [3] and mental health [4]. More precisely, there is increasing evidence of the adverse health effects of excessive sedentary behaviour [5–7]. This evidence is mainly seen for common sedentary behaviours, such as screen time (e.g., TV viewing, video game playing, computer use) and sitting time (e.g., riding in automobiles, reading). Taking this evidence into account, for the first time in 2020, the World Health Organization issued global recommendations for sedentary time alongside physical activity recommendations [1]. These recommendations state that the amount of time spent sedentary should be limited, particularly recreational screen time, and replaced with physical activity of any intensity.

As an emerging research topic, methods of assessing sedentary behaviour have advanced significantly in recent years, from the refinement of self-report measures to the swift advances of device-based measurement [8]. These adequate methods have helped better understand sedentary behaviour's accumulation patterns and contexts, determinants and associations. Notwithstanding, new evidence on sedentary behaviour is ever-growing. The complementarity of evidence regarding sedentary behaviour measurement, mechanisms, and interventions should be emphasized to inform public health guidelines and policy better [8].

The study of sedentary behaviour is of importance, now more than ever. As our knowledge of this behaviour is rapidly advancing, more questions arise. Therefore, there is still room to grow and avenues to explore for developing and refining the understanding of sedentary behaviour. Thus, this book contributes to better understanding of sedentary behaviour and its health implications, both in Western countries and in some countries in epidemiological transition, such as those in sub-Saharan Africa. It contains the current definitions of sedentary behaviour and the various methods used for its measurement and evaluation. As sedentary behaviour is a risk factor for health, it is essential to understand the benefits of its constant interruption, especially in reducing the risk of cardiovascular disease. This book intends to make a small contribution in these areas, presenting the reader with recent scientific evidence.

Adilson Marques
Faculdade de Motricidade Humana,
Universidade de Lisboa,
Lisboa, Portugal

Élvio Rúbio Gouveia
Universidade da Madeira,
Funchal, Portugal

References

[1] Bull FC, Al-Ansari SS, Biddle S, Borodulin K, Buman MP, Cardon G, et al. World Health Organization 2020 guidelines on physical activity and sedentary behaviour. Br J Sports Med. 2020;**54**(24):1451-62.

[2] Bailey DP, Hewson DJ, Champion RB, Sayegh SM. Sitting Time and Risk of Cardiovascular Disease and Diabetes: A Systematic Review and Meta-Analysis. Am J Prev Med. 2019;**57**(3):408-16.

[3] Schmid D, Leitzmann MF. Television viewing and time spent sedentary in relation to cancer risk: a meta-analysis. J Natl Cancer Inst. 2014;**106**(7).

[4] Zhai L, Zhang Y, Zhang D. Sedentary behaviour and the risk of depression: a meta-analysis. Br J Sports Med. 2015;**49**(11):705-9.

[5] Patterson R, McNamara E, Tainio M, de Sa TH, Smith AD, Sharp SJ, et al. Sedentary behaviour and risk of all-cause, cardiovascular and cancer mortality, and incident type 2 diabetes: a systematic review and dose response meta-analysis. Eur J Epidemiol. 2018;**33**(9):811-29.

[6] Katzmarzyk PT, Powell KE, Jakicic JM, Troiano RP, Piercy K, Tennant B, et al. Sedentary Behavior and Health: Update from the 2018 Physical Activity Guidelines Advisory Committee. Med Sci Sports Exerc. 2019;**51**(6):1227-41.

[7] Biswas A, Oh PI, Faulkner GE, Bajaj RR, Silver MA, Mitchell MS, et al. Sedentary time and its association with risk for disease incidence, mortality, and hospitalization in adults: a systematic review and meta-analysis. Ann Intern Med. 2015;**162**(2):123-32.

[8] Owen N, Healy GN, Dempsey PC, Salmon J, Timperio A, Clark BK, et al. Sedentary Behavior and Public Health: Integrating the Evidence and Identifying Potential Solutions. Annu Rev Public Health. 2020;**41**:265-87.

Chapter 1

Sedentary Behaviour: Definition, Determinants, Impacts on Health, and Current Recommendations

Priscila Marconcin, Vera Zymbal, Élvio R. Gouveia, Bruce Jones and Adilson Marques

Abstract

This chapter aims to present an overview of the scientific background and current recommendations for sedentary behaviour. We have presented the current sedentary behaviour definition and defined other terms related to sedentary behaviour. The determinants of sedentary behaviour were discussed, and the ecological model was presented. Based on the recent data from the literature, the relationship between sedentary behaviour and health indicators was presented and discussed. Finally, we discussed the recommendation regarding sedentary behaviour, and presented the daily guidelines involving physical activity, sedentary behaviour, and sleep routine.

Keywords: sedentary behaviour definition, physically inactive, health outcomes, sedentary behaviour determinants, 24-hour guidelines

1. Introduction

Sedentary behaviour (SB) is a health risk independent of age, population, sex, or clinical condition [1, 2]. Evidence highlights a negative association of prolonged sedentary time, and patterns of sedentary time, with cardio-metabolic risk biomarkers and health outcomes [1, 3]. However, studies in recent years have presented inconsistency related to the sedentary behaviour definition. This has made some difficulties for studies in the field itself [4]. This chapter clarifies SB definition based on the information from the Sedentary Behaviour Research Network (SBRN).

A comprehensive research agenda on SB also includes measurement studies, and evaluating the outcomes of environmental and policy initiatives. The conceptual basis for these studies includes an ecological model of behavioural determinants [5]. These models recognise how individual behaviours are affected by environmental and policy factors [5]. This conceptualisation of SB leads to explicit consideration of multiple complex levels of influence, such as: intrapersonal (biological, psychological), interpersonal (social, cultural), organisational, community, and physical environment.

This chapter aims to contribute to the existing evidence, and to clarify and discuss the following important aspects of SB: the current definition, the definition of related terms, the determinants of SB, the relationship between SB and health outcomes, and the current guidelines worldwide regarding SB. We expect to contribute to public health initiatives designed to develop more feasible interventions that focus on diminishing SB among all age groups.

2. Definition of sedentary behaviour

Society has encountered rapid and significant physical, economic, and social environment changes, leading to increased inactivity among individuals in the workplace, in transportation, in communication, and at home. These changes have had significant negative consequences on health-related behaviours.

The study of sedentary behaviour (SB) started with a study by Morris and colleagues in 1953. They investigated bus drivers and desk-bound workers in the United Kingdom, concluding that those who were more active presented significantly reduced cardiovascular disease risk than those who were less active [6]. Although these findings refer to the level of physical activity (PA), it can be speculated that SB was also a relevant factor that should have been assessed [7].

As interest in SB research has increased, what has emerged is a lack of consistency and agreement in SB, as well as the definition of related terms. Over the past few decades, the term "sedentary" has been used in different ways (e.g., to define those who do little or no PA, or those who do not fulfil the PA guidelines) [8]. The SB definition has been based on two aspects: postural and energy expenditure. SB has been generally defined as the time spent in a sitting or reclining posture. This definition stems from the Latin origin of the word sedentary, *sedere* (to sit). From the energy expenditure aspect, SB is usually defined as the time spent in any waking behaviour that requires low levels of energy expenditure (e.g. ≤1.5 METs).

Although postural and energy expenditure aspects are crucial to determine SB, research in this field typically includes only one of these components. One of the reasons is related to the methods used to measure SB. Assessment methods of SB include subjective and objective measurements, each one providing different information. Studies analysing SB from the postural aspect usually employ questionnaires, direct observation, or inclinometers, The energy expenditure aspect is commonly estimated indirectly by accelerometry. In contrast with these aspects, many studies described their participants as sedentary when they did not achieve a recommended amount of PA. The variety of measurement methods, and conflicting definitions of SB, has generated misunderstanding, making it difficult to not only compare studies, but also to understand the real impact of SB on health outcomes. Consequently, researchers have begun to call for clearer and more precise definitions and measurements [9].

To prevent contradiction and consternation, in 2012, the Sedentary Behaviour Research Network (SBRN), an organisation of researchers and health professionals, published a letter to define the differences between "sedentary behaviour" and "physical inactivity" [10]. In this first consensus publication, the SBRN suggested that SB should be defined "*as any waking behaviour characterised by an energy expenditure ≤ 1.5 metabolic equivalents (METs), while in a sitting or reclining posture*" [10]. This definition included both postural (sitting or reclining), and energy expenditure (<1.5 METS) aspects. In addition, the term "inactive" should be used to describe those who "*...are performing insufficient amounts of moderate to vigorous PA (i.e. not meeting specified PA guidelines)*" [10]. According to these terms, a person can be active when meeting PA guidelines, but also spend a large amount of their day in SB.

The distinction between SB and physical inactivity terms has provided important progress on the SB field. However, there remains a need to refine, and establish a consensus for, various other SB terms (e.g., screen time, sedentary behaviour pattern, bouts, and breaks). Moreover, some terms were considered inappropriate when applied to different age categories (e.g. infants, before learning to sit and stand) or populations with different physical capacities (e.g. people with mobility impairment). In this context, the SBRN developed a project to provide a consensus definition for terms related to SB research for all age groups and all physical abilities. The results were published in 2017 [4] and define several concepts related to SB.

Sedentary behaviour. General population: Any waking behaviour characterised by an energy expenditure ≤1.5 metabolic equivalents (METs), while in a sitting, reclining, or lying posture [10]. Infants (<1 year or pre-walking): Any waking behaviour characterised by low energy expenditure while restrained or when calm. Time spent in the prone position ("tummy time") is not considered a sedentary exposure.

Sedentary time. The time spent for any duration or in any context in sedentary behaviours.
Sedentary bout. A period of uninterrupted sedentary time.
Sedentary interruptions/breaks. A non-sedentary bout in between two sedentary bouts.

Physical inactivity. Insufficient PA level to meet present PA recommendations [11, 12].

Stationary behaviour. Any waking behaviour performed while lying, reclining, sitting, or standing, with no ambulation, irrespective of energy expenditure. This definition applies to all age and ability groups except infants.

Stationary time. The time spent in stationary behaviours.
Stationary bout. A period of uninterrupted stationary time.
Stationary interruptions/breaks. A non-stationary bout in between two stationary bouts.

Standing, A position in which one has or is maintaining an upright position while supported by one's feet.

Active standing. Any activity in a standing posture characterised by an energy expenditure >2.0 METs, while standing without ambulation, whether supported or unsupported.
Passive standing. Any standing position without ambulation characterised by an energy expenditure ≤2.0 METs.
Standing time. The time spent for any duration or in any context while standing.
Standing bout. A period of uninterrupted time while standing.
Standing breaks. A non-standing bout in between two standing bouts.

Screen Time. Time spent on screen-based behaviours [13, 14]. These behaviours can be performed while being sedentary or physically active.

Recreational screen time. Time spent in screen behaviours that are not related to school or work [15].
Stationary screen time. Time spent using a screen-based device while being stationary in any context.
Sedentary screen time. Time spent using a screen-based device while being sedentary in any context.
Active screen time. Time spent using a screen-based device while not being stationary in any context.

Non-screen-based sedentary time. Refers to the time spent in sedentary behaviours that do not involve the use of screens.

Sitting. A position in which one's weight is supported by one's buttocks rather than one's feet, and in which one's back is upright.

Active sitting. Any waking activity in a sitting posture characterised by an energy expenditure >1.5 METs.
Passive sitting. Any waking activity in a sitting posture characterised by an energy expenditure ≤1.5 METs.

Reclining. Reclining is a body position between sitting and lying.

Active reclining. >1.5 METs.
Passive reclining. ≤ 1.5 METs.

Lying. Refers to being in a horizontal position on a supporting surface.

Active lying. >1.5 METs.
Passive lying. ≤ 1.5 METs.

Sedentary behaviour pattern. It is how sedentary behaviour is accumulated throughout the day or week while awake [16, 17].

In summary, the definition of SB and related terms has evolved. Currently, much progress has been made. However, studies are needed to validate the proposed terms. Also, much discussion still exists about MET values thresholds, and future studies are needed to determine values that best represent SB at different ages, and physical and health conditions. Also, standardisation of assessment and analysis of SB by accelerometry is necessary.

Difference between physical activity and sedentary behaviour.

To reduce the risk of developing chronic disease, and to maintain a healthy lifestyle, public health interventions focus on improving PA and reducing SB. Despite both constructs being similar in their objectives, they present differences regarding interventions that should be highlighted. These relate mainly to the frequency and duration of the two behaviours. Interventions on PA usually aim to encourage participants to accumulate more moderate to vigorous PA (MVPA). Interventions on SB are designed to support people to shift some of their sedentary time to light intensity activities [18]. It is essential to highlight the difference between being inactive and being sedentary. Inactive individuals present low/insufficient levels of MVPA, while sedentary individuals show a high level of sitting [19]. It is possible, for example, to be highly active (go to the gym five times a week for one hour) and sedentary (work in an office setting for more than 6 hours, without break times).

To standardise the PA intensity, in the late 1980s, the Compendium of PA was developed and was updated in 2011 [20]. The Compendium standardises the MET (metabolic equivalent) intensities used in a variety of PA. It does not correct the MET levels for age, body mass, and gender. The Physical Activity Guidelines Advisory Committee [21] defined PA intensity as:

Light-intensity activity *is non-sedentary waking behaviour that requires less than 3.0 METs; examples include walking at a slow or leisurely pace (2 mph or less), cooking activities, or light household chores.*
Moderate-intensity activity *requires 3.0 to less than 6.0 METs; examples include walking briskly (2.5 to 4 mph), playing doubles tennis, or raking the yard.*

> **Vigorous-intensity activity** *requires 6.0 or more METs; examples include jogging, running, carrying heavy groceries or other loads upstairs, shovelling snow, or participating in a strenuous fitness class.*

This guideline was updated in 2018, but the intensity defined for energy expended was maintained. Through the guidelines, four levels of aerobic PA were made: inactive, insufficiently active, active, and highly active [22].

> **Inactive** *is not getting any moderate- or vigorous-intensity PA beyond basic movement from daily life activities.*
> **Insufficiently active** *is doing some moderate- or vigorous-intensity PA but less than 150 minutes of moderate-intensity PA a week or 75 minutes of vigorous-intensity PA or the equivalent combination. This level is less than the target range for meeting the key guidelines for adults.*
> **Active** *is doing the equivalent of 150 minutes to 300 minutes of moderate-intensity PA a week. This level meets the key guideline target range for adults.*
> **Highly active** *is doing the equivalent of more than 300 minutes of moderate-intensity PA a week. This level exceeds the key guideline target range for adults.*

This classification of PA intensity is the same as the one used by the World Health Organisation to make guidelines regarding PA and health for adults [23]. The difference between SB and PA is critical to recognising the distinct determinants of SB and PA, and to designing public health interventions that are most suitable. Interventions focusing on SB should not follow the same approach used for PA interventions. They must be more specific and must emphasise SB's determinants.

3. Determinants of sedentary behaviour

It is essential to comprehend the modifiable determinants of PA and SB, and to translate that knowledge into practical actions to benefit public health. The simple cause and effect pathway of health behaviours (e.g. SB and health outcomes) is an unwise approach to take. Motivating or educating individuals to change their behaviour is likely to be restricted if their physical and socio-cultural environments do not enable and support the behaviour [24].

3.1 Ecological model of sedentary behaviour

The ecological approach considers multiple levels of influence on a specific behaviour, such as: individual, social, organisational/community, environmental, and public policy [25]. The ecological model distinguishes itself from individual-level models by focusing on the interaction of person-level attributes (e.g. motivation, self-efficacy) with physical and socio-cultural environments [26]. Ecological models have been used to explore and address several different health behaviours (e.g. PA, healthy eating, and tobacco smoking) [25]. Regarding SB, it is crucial to understand which physical attribute is in focus, and the context in which the SB occurs. The ecological model of SB, highlighting the influence of particular contexts or domains in which behaviours occur, considers four domains: leisure, household, transport, and occupation [5]. Each domain presents a range of potential influences.

The key of the Ecological Model of SB is to understand which social and environmental factors could influence the SB. Various factors are likely to influence an individual's choice and risk of engaging in SB. Also, it is important to consider the population target and the settings. For example, for working adults with sedentary jobs, making changes in the workplace must diminish SB at the workplace [27]. The Torbeyns et al. study concluded that a standing desk intervention increase the HDL cholesterol, and decrease postprandial glucose when compared with a seated workstation [28]. For older adults and retirees, SB's main setting is in the home. Interventions should therefore focus on this setting [29]. For children and adolescents, it is important to look for the main SB, which is screen viewing in different settings [30]. Also, there are some SB's that occur in a specific setting, which must be considered. For example, TV viewing frequently occurs at home. This correlation is important for the purpose of targeting an intervention focused on the setting, beyond the behaviour. Understanding SB's correlates in a specific setting is thus important to develop more effective interventions [5]. Workplace furniture is growing in popularity as an intervention tool for the purpose of decreasing SB. For example, employees with long-term access to sit-stand desks sit less, and sit upright more often, than employees with sitting desks [31]. **Figure 1** shows the variables that could be studied for each domain.

A systematic review among adults aged 18–65 years found seventy-four studies that aimed to identify individual, social, environmental, and policy-related determinants or correlates of SB [32]. The results indicated that individual-level factors (e.g. age, PA levels, body mass index, socioeconomic status, and mood) were significantly correlated with SB. A trend towards increased leisure screen time was identified in those married or cohabiting, while having children resulted in less total sitting time. Also, the proximity of green space, neighbourhood walkability and safety, weather, and other environmental factors were correlated with SB [32]. Although this systematic review is an important contribution to the SB field, most included studies were observational. No longitudinal study was performed, which makes it difficult to make a causal inference. Only longitudinal studies allow for the establishment of a causal relationship.

Another systematic review conducted to better understand factors associated with SB among older adults found twenty-two high quality studies (median of 82%, IQR 69–96%, using Qualsyst tool), almost all of which were cross-sectional and observational [33]. Their results showed older and retired individuals were seated often. Some studies considered environmental determinants. This conclusion suggests a possible association with mode of transport, type of housing, cultural opportunities, neighbourhood safety, and availability of places to rest [33]. However, the systematic review included only studies from high-income countries. More evidence is needed from lower- and middle-income countries. In addition, there is minimal causal evidence for the association of environmental determinants

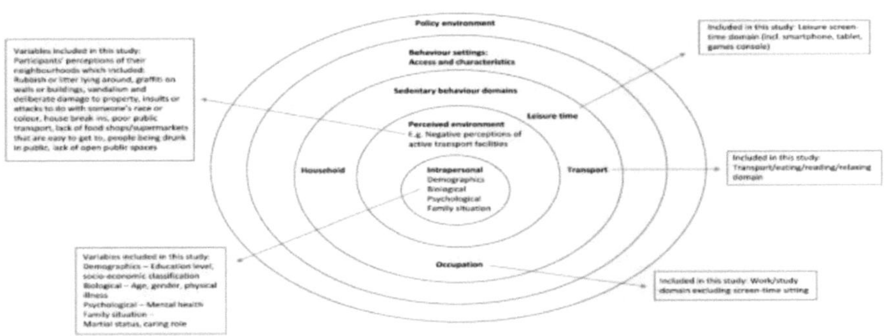

Figure 1.
Mapping of the domains and correlated variables of the ecological model of sedentary behaviour. Published on Nicolson, Hayes [24] with permission.

and sedentary behaviour, as the vast majority of information comes from quantitative cross-sectional studies. Longitudinal and experimental approaches would be necessary to identify potential levels that could be used to design innovative interventions, for older adults, to diminish the SB.

Among youth, more studies are available. Stierlin et al. reviewed thirty-seven studies; only high quality longitudinal, intervention, and observational studies were included (median of 82%, IQR: 74–91%, using the Qualsyst tool) [34]. Determinants were found at the individual, interpersonal, environmental, and public policy levels. Age and weight status were positively associated with total SB. Also, baseline assessment of screen time was positively associated with screen time at follow-up. A higher playground density, and higher availability of play and sports equipment at school, was consistently related to an increased total SB, although these consistent findings come from single studies. Other study reported the association of the proximity of safe places to crossroads, and lengthening morning and lunch breaks, with less total SB [34].

All cited systematic reviews were essential to a better understanding of the determinants of SB. However, across the studies, we learn more about the "who" of SB engagement, and less about the "why" of their SB engagement. To make substantial advancements in intervention design, and to gain insights into important and modifiable mediators of behavioural change, researchers need to know the motivational and contextual reasons for engaging in SB [35]. Information about the various levels and types of influences and contributors to SB may help develop multi-level interventions that expand the chances to decrease sedentary behaviour. More studies, focusing specifically on motivation, abilities, and opportunities, as well as unconscious processes that may induce and sustain changes in SB, are crucial [35].

4. Sedentary behaviour and health

Sedentary behaviour has been a big concern of public health and prevention medicine. Over the last decades, a growing interest has been placed on the health impact of SB. Wise public health recommendations about SB can only be made if there is a clear understanding of its relationship with various health impacts. In this respect, many studies have shown that higher amounts of SB are associated with harmful health outcomes such as metabolic syndrome, obesity, diabetes, cardiovascular diseases, and mortality [1, 3].

The Physical Activity Guidelines Advisory Committee Scientific Report (PAGAC) provided an overview of relationships between SB and mortality; it exposed the weight status of SB among several non-communicable diseases [36]. The conclusion was that there was strong evidence that high amounts of SB increase the risk for all-cause and cardiovascular disease (CVD) mortality, also incident CVD and type 2 diabetes. In addition, it showed, with moderate evidence, that SB was associated with incident endometrial, colon, and lung cancer. There was limited evidence which demonstrated that SB was associated with cancer mortality and weight control. Considering PA status, the study concluded that SB's hazardous effects are more pronounced in physically inactive participants [36]. A prospective cohort study showed that greater sedentary time was associated with all-cause mortality [37].

Along with the relationship between SB and mortality, it is important to analyse other health parameters such as: pain, quality of life, mental health, function and disability. An overview, of systematic reviews that examined the relationship between SB and a range of health indicators among the adult population, was done in 2020. The main findings are summarised in **Table 1** [51].

Outcome	Studies (systematic reviews)	Main findings
Health-related quality of life (HRQOL)	Boberska et al. (2018) Castro et al. (2018) Ramalho et al. (2018)	Higher levels of SB are associated with lower physical HRQoL [38]. Total screen time was negatively associated with social quality of life. There were no significant associations observed between SB and environmental, personal, or overall quality of life [39]. Significant and negative associations between SB and quality of life [40].
Brain health	Falck et al. (2017)	The odds of developing Alzheimer's increased 1.32 (95% CI: 1.08, 1.62) for each 1-h increase in daily TV viewing [41].
Cognitive function (CF)	Falck et al. (2017) Castro et al. (2018) Ramalho et al. (2018) Sui et al. (2019)	Negative associations between SB and CF [41]. Executive function was negatively associated with total sedentary time. Working memory capacity was not associated with self-reported sitting, screen time, or passive transportation. And, perceived cognitive ability was negatively associated with total sitting time, but not associated with device-measured sedentary time [39]. CF was negatively associated with TV viewing. CF was positively associated with Internet/ computer use. CF was not associated with device-measured sitting [40]. No difference between seated and non-seated workstations, non-seated workstations were associated with improved cognitive performance, and non-seated workstations were associated with reduced cognitive performance [42].
Depression	Zhai et al. (2015) Teychenne et al. (2010) Ramalho et al. (2018)	Participants reporting high SB had a 1.14 (95% CI: 1.06, 1.21) relative risk of depression [43]. Positive associations between SB and depression or depressive symptoms. Total sedentary time and TV viewing were generally positively associated with depression or depressive symptoms, while Internet and computer use often demonstrated beneficial associations with depression or depressive symptoms [44]. 4/6 studies observed null associations between SB and depressive symptoms [40].
Musculoskeletal pain	Castro et al. (2018) Shrestha et al. (2018) Josaphat et al. (2019)	Positive associations were observed between musculoskeletal symptoms and a total sitting time (3/3 studies), computer use (8/10 studies), video games (1/3 studies), and mobile phones (2/6 studies). No associations were observed between musculoskeletal symptoms and TV viewing (1/1 studies), total screen time (1/1 studies), or studying (3/3 studies) [39]. Lower prevalence of musculoskeletal symptoms in participants using sit-stand desks when compared with sit-desks [45]. Reduced discomfort when alternating sitting and standing when compared with sitting for 8 h [46].

Outcome	Studies (systematic reviews)	Main findings
Accidents and injuries	O'Donoghue et al. (2016) Rezende et al. (2014) Shrestha et al. (2018)	No association between self-reported sitting time (n = 4) or device- measured sedentary time (n = 1) and disability, illness, or injury. A positive association between transport sitting time and disability, illness, or injury [32]. No eligible studies were identified [47]. Excluding the musculoskeletal pain described previously, no adverse events were reported [45].
Biomarkers of cardiometabolic risk	Torbeyns et al. (2014) Wirth et al. (2017) Josaphat et al. (2019) Saunders et al. (2018)	Standing desk intervention reported an increase in HDL cholesterol, and a decrease in postprandial glucose, when compared with a seated workstation, treadmill desk intervention reported a significant reduction in total and LDL-cholesterol [28]. Significant reduction in fasting insulin levels in favour of the intervention group (targeting reduced SB), with no changes observed for total, HDL- or LDL cholesterol, or fasting glucose [48]. Standing workstations resulted in improved measures of glycaemic control when compared with seated workstations (3/4 studies). Treadmill workstations resulted in lower HbA1c levels (2/3 studies). Improved total and LDL-cholesterol levels (1/3 studies). Improvements in HDL cholesterol (1/3 studies). No changes in cholesterol levels (1/3 studies). No changes in fasting insulin, glucose, or triglycerides in response to treadmill desk use (3/3 studies) [46]. Breaking up sitting time was associated with benefits in postprandial glucose [49].
Body composition	Neuhaus et al. (2014) Josaphat et al. (2019) Wirth et al. (2017)	Significant improvement in waist circumference (3/3 studies using a treadmill or pedal desk). Reported no change (2/2 studies using sit-stand desk). Significant improvement in BMI following the introduction of an activity permissive workstation (1 study) [50]. Significant improvement in at least 1 measure of body composition (3/3 studies using a treadmill desk). 2/2 randomised studies failed to detect any changes in body composition. 2/2 randomised studies using a sit-stand desk reported no change in body composition [46]. No change in waist circumference (1/1intervention study targeting reduced SB in older adults) [48].

Abbreviation: BMI, body mass index; CF, cardiorespiratory fitness; CI, confidence interval; HDL, high-density lipoprotein; HRQoL, health-related quality of life; LDL, low-density lipoprotein; SB, sedentary behaviour; TV, television.

Table 1.
Overview of systematic review regarding the relationship between SB and a range of health indicators among the adult population. Adapted from Saunders et al. [21].

Another important consideration about SB's impact on health is the relationship between different elements of SB, such as bouts, frequency, duration, and timing. The PAGAC Scientific Report (2018) showed insufficient evidence to determine if bout length or breaks in sedentary behaviour are associated with health outcomes [36]. However, other studies suggest that SB patterns may be associated with an increased risk of mortality, among other health outcomes. Longer mean sedentary bout duration was associated with all-cause mortality [37]. Prolonged sitting resulted in moderate elevations in postprandial glucose and insulin responses when compared to sitting interrupted with activity breaks [49, 52]. Also, the sedentary break on sitting behaviour was associated to attenuate cardiometabolic risk markers [53].

5. Guidelines and recommendation of sedentary behaviour

There is a global consensus regarding the need to reduce SB, but some questions still need to be clarified. How much sedentary time might be unsafe or detrimental to health? How frequently should SB be broken up, and what type and intensity of PA would be desirable in doing so?

For the first time, in November 2020, the World Health Organisation (WHO) provided evidence-based public health recommendations on the amount of PA, in association with SB, to offer health benefits and mitigate health risk [54]. It was the first time that SB has appeared in a WHO guideline. Although it was a significant step forward, the recommendation falls short with respect to specificity; it did not provide a threshold of SB or sedentary time. The WHO guideline is intended for policy-makers in high-middle and low-income countries, and in ministries of health, education, youth, sport, and/or social or family welfare. Local authorities should be responsible for elaborate feasible plans to improve PA and reduce SB. In this sense, the recommendations are a good step.

In a national setting, Canada was the first country to make specific recommendations regarding SB and screen time for adults and older adults [55]. The guidelines follow the 24-hour SB Research Network movement guidelines [4]. A systematic review provided evidence that the daily movement behaviour composition was associated with health outcomes, such as adiposity and cardiometabolic biomarkers, in addition to being associated with all-cause mortality [56]. Also, reallocating time into other movement behaviour from SB was associated with positive changes to all-cause mortality [56].

The Canadian 24-Hour Movement Guidelines for Adults aged 18–64 years, and Adults aged 65 years or older, integrates recommendations for a healthy day (24 h) comprised of a combination of PA, SB, and sleep. The guidelines were generated based on the best available evidence, and should be updated every 10 years (or whenever important new evidence is identified that could inform and/or suggest revisions to the existing guideline recommendations). The guidelines are for adults (18–64 years) and older adults (65 years or older), irrespective of gender, cultural background, or socioeconomic status. The exceptions to the guidelines are for pregnant women or persons living with a disability or medical condition. The guidelines recognise that individuals should be engaged in different PA during the day (e.g. weight bearing/non-weight bearing, sport, and recreation) in a variety of environments (e.g. home/work/community; indoor/outdoor, land/water) and contexts (e.g. leisure, transportation, occupation, household). Moreover, the guidelines highlight that adults should limit long periods of SB and should practice healthy sleep hygiene. For adults, a healthy 24-hours includes; (1) PA (150 minutes per week of moderate to vigorous aerobic PA, twice a week of muscle strength and several hours of light PA, including standing); (2) sleep (7–9 hours of good quality sleep); (3) SB (limited to 8 hours or less, no more than 3 hours' recreation screen time and breaking up long periods of SB as often as possible. Also, the guidelines suggest replacing SB with additional PA and trading light PA for more moderate to vigorous PA. The difference in the guidelines for older adults regards the addition of PA, beyond the adult recommendation, that addresses balance [55].

The breakthrough of the Canadian 24-Hour Movement Guidelines was that, for the first time, guidelines identify specific threshold values for daily SB and recreational screen time. The value was based on meta-analyses which suggested that the risk of all-cause mortality increased more rapidly above the threshold value range from 7 to 9.5 h/day for daily SB [1, 57]. Self-reported measures had a lower threshold when compared to device-based measures of SB. Concerning screen-based SB studies, there was a variety of thresholds that increased the risk of all-cause mortality (i.e., 3 h/day [57, 58], 3.5 h/day [1], and 4 h/day of TV viewing [59]). The authors found that it would be impractical to provide a range of thresholds, indicating that 8 h/day of SB and 3 h/day of TV viewing would be most appropriate.

Before these guidelines, in 2017, Canada had already developed 24-h movement guidelines for early years (0–4 years) [11] and children and youth (5–17 years) [15]. Other countries also follow the same principle, and have presented 24-h movement guidelines for children up to 5 years of age, including Australia [60], New Zealand [61], and South Africa [62]. In 2019, the WHO presented similar recommendations for 24-hour PA, sedentary behaviour, and sleep for children under the age of 5 [63].

6. Conclusion

In our technological society, people progressively change their behaviour, increasing the time spent in activities with low energy expenditure. This change in behaviour has had a significant impact on public health. Currently, studies have associated excessive SB with adverse health outcomes. Therefore, to better comprehend the relationship between health outcomes and sedentary behaviour, and to make advancements in this field, it is essential to present a standardised operational definition of SB and related terms. The Sedentary Behaviour Research Network (SBRN) coordinated a comprehensive effort to develop further consensus definitions for terms related to SB. We have presented, in a table, a summary of this information. The standardisation of research, in the SB field, is vital.

It is critical to understand which factors influence SB among children, adolescents, adults, and older adults. The ecological model of SB presents an approach that considers multiple levels of influences, while addressing four main domains in which SB can occur (each sharing similar characteristics). These domains are: leisure, household, transport, and occupation. Research in the SB field must consider individual factors, and their interaction with environmental factors, in each of these domains (and for each age group).

This chapter provided data from current studies that investigated the association between SB and different health outcomes, such as: health-related quality of life, brain health, cognitive function, depression, musculoskeletal pain, accidents and injuries, biomarkers of cardiometabolic risk, and body composition. Beyond that, we discussed SB's association with all-cause mortality, while considering such elements as total time, bouts, frequency, and intensity.

Finally, we presented the World Health Organisation guidelines regarding PA in association with SB. The last guidelines, from 2020, did not provide a threshold of SB, but national ones, from Canada, provided guidelines based on the 24-hour model, dividing the recommendation into PA, sleep and SB, while offering, for the first time, a specific time-limit for SB and screen recreation time.

With this current information, we expect to help researchers to make advancements in the SB field. More studies are needed, not only to provide specific guidelines considering the bouts, frequency, and intensity of SB, but also to better understand the association between SB bouts and all-cause mortality. Experimental studies are needed on: the dose–response relationships and underlying mechanisms of SB and health outcomes, the feasibility of changing prolonged sedentary time, how best to promote maintenance of the relevant SB changes, and the health benefits to be realised.

Author details

Priscila Marconcin[1*], Vera Zymbal[1], Élvio R. Gouveia[2], Bruce Jones[3] and Adilson Marques[1]

1 Faculty of Human Kinetics, University of Lisbon, Lisbon, Portugal

2 University of Madeira, Funchal, Portugal

3 Queen's University, Kingston, Canada

*Address all correspondence to: priscilamarconcin@fmh.ulisboa.pt

References

[1] Patterson R, McNamara E, Tainio M, de Sá TH, Smith AD, Sharp SJ, et al. Sedentary behaviour and risk of all-cause, cardiovascular and cancer mortality, and incident type 2 diabetes: a systematic review and dose response meta-analysis. European journal of epidemiology. 2018;33(9):811-829.

[2] Fenton SAM, Veldhuijzen van Zanten JJCS, Kitas GD, Duda JL, Rouse PC, Yu C-a, et al. Sedentary behaviour is associated with increased long-term cardiovascular risk in patients with rheumatoid arthritis independently of moderate-to-vigorous physical activity. BMC Musculoskeletal Disorders. 2017;18(1):131.

[3] Lemes I, Sui X, Fernandes R, Blair S, Turi-Lynch B, Codogno J, et al. Association of sedentary behavior and metabolic syndrome. Public Health. 2019;167:96-102.

[4] Tremblay MS, Aubert S, Barnes JD, Saunders TJ, Carson V, Latimer-Cheung AE, et al. Sedentary Behavior Research Network (SBRN) – Terminology Consensus Project process and outcome. International Journal of Behavioral Nutrition and Physical Activity. 2017;14(1):75.

[5] Owen N, Sugiyama T, Eakin EE, Gardiner PA, Tremblay MS, Sallis JF. Adults' Sedentary Behavior: Determinants and Interventions. American journal of preventive medicine. 2011;41(2):189-196.

[6] Morris JN, Crawford MD. Coronary heart disease and physical activity of work; evidence of a national necropsy survey. Br Med J. 1958;2(5111): 1485-1496.

[7] Zhu W, Owen N. Sedentary behavior and health: Concepts, assessments, and interventions: Human Kinetics; 2017.

[8] Owen N, Healy GN, Matthews CE, Dunstan DW. Too much sitting: the population health science of sedentary behavior. Exerc Sport Sci Rev. 2010; 38(3):105-113.

[9] Yates T, Wilmot EG, Davies MJ, Gorely T, Edwardson C, Biddle S, et al. Sedentary behavior: what's in a definition? American journal of preventive medicine. 2011;40(6):e33-4; author reply e4.

[10] Network SBR. Letter to the editor: standardized use of the terms "sedentary" and "sedentary behaviours". Applied physiology, nutrition, and metabolism = Physiologie appliquee, nutrition et metabolisme. 2012;37(3): 540-2.

[11] Tremblay MS, Chaput JP, Adamo KB, Aubert S, Barnes JD, Choquette L, et al. Canadian 24-hour movement guidelines for the early years (0-4 years): an integration of physical activity, sedentary behaviour, and sleep. BMC public health. 2017;17(Suppl 5): 874.

[12] Lee IM, Shiroma EJ, Lobelo F, Puska P, Blair SN, Katzmarzyk PT. Effect of physical inactivity on major non-communicable diseases worldwide: an analysis of burden of disease and life expectancy. Lancet (London, England). 2012;380(9838):219-29.

[13] Stamatakis E, Hamer M, Dunstan DW. Screen-based entertainment time, all-cause mortality, and cardiovascular events: population-based study with ongoing mortality and hospital events follow-up. Journal of the American College of Cardiology. 2011;57(3):292-299.

[14] Anderson SE, Economos CD, Must A. Active play and screen time in US children aged 4 to 11 years in relation to sociodemographic and weight status characteristics: a nationally

representative cross-sectional analysis. BMC public health. 2008;8(1):366.

[15] Tremblay MS, Carson V, Chaput JP, Connor Gorber S, Dinh T, Duggan M, et al. Canadian 24-hour movement guidelines for children and youth: an integration of physical activity, sedentary behaviour, and sleep. Appl Physiol Nutr Metab. 2016;41 (6 Suppl 3):S311-S327.

[16] Chastin SF, Granat MH. Methods for objective measure, quantification and analysis of sedentary behaviour and inactivity. Gait & posture. 2010;31(1):82-86.

[17] Chinapaw MJM, de Niet M, Verloigne M, De Bourdeaudhuij I, Brug J, Altenburg TM. From sedentary time to sedentary patterns: accelerometer data reduction decisions in youth. PloS one. 2014;9(11): e111205-e.

[18] Hadgraft NT, Dunstan DW, Owen N. Models for Understanding Sedentary Behaviour. In: Leitzmann MF, Jochem C, Schmid D, editors. Sedentary Behaviour Epidemiology. Cham: Springer International Publishing; 2018. p. 381-403.

[19] Lynch BM, Healy GN, Dunstan DW, Owen N. Sedentary versus inactive: distinctions for disease prevention. Nature reviews Cardiology. 2010;7(11):doi:10.1083/nrcardio. 2010.68-c1; author reply doi:10.1083/ nrcardio.2010.68-c2.

[20] Ainsworth BE, Haskell WL, Herrmann SD, Meckes N, Bassett DR, Jr., Tudor-Locke C, et al. 2011 Compendium of Physical Activities: a second update of codes and MET values. Medicine and science in sports and exercise. 2011;43(8):1575-1581.

[21] Physical Activity Guidelines Advisory Committee. Physical Activity Guidelines Advisory Committee report, 2008. Washington, DC: U.S. Department of Health and Human Services; 2008.

[22] Piercy KL, Troiano RP, Ballard RM, Carlson SA, Fulton JE, Galuska DA, et al. The Physical Activity Guidelines for Americans. Jama. 2018;320(19): 2020-2028.

[23] Bull FC, Al-Ansari SS, Biddle S, Borodulin K, Buman MP, Cardon G, et al. World Health Organization 2020 guidelines on physical activity and sedentary behaviour. British journal of sports medicine. 2020;54(24):1451.

[24] Nicolson G, Hayes C, Darker C. Examining total and domain-specific sedentary behaviour using the socio-ecological model – a cross-sectional study of Irish adults. BMC public health. 2019;19(1):1155.

[25] Sallis JF, Owen N, Fisher E. Ecological models of health behavior. Health behavior: Theory, research, and practice. 2015;5(43-64).

[26] Stokols D, Grzywacz JG, McMahan S, Phillips K. Increasing the health promotive capacity of human environments. American journal of health promotion : AJHP. 2003;18(1): 4-13.

[27] Bennie JA, Pedisic Z, Timperio A, Crawford D, Dunstan D, Bauman A, et al. Total and domain-specific sitting time among employees in desk-based work settings in Australia. Australian and New Zealand journal of public health. 2015;39(3):237-242.

[28] Torbeyns T, Bailey S, Bos I, Meeusen R. Active workstations to fight sedentary behaviour. Sports medicine (Auckland, NZ). 2014;44(9):1261-73.

[29] Harvey JA, Chastin SFM, Skelton DA. Prevalence of sedentary behavior in older adults: a systematic review. International journal of

environmental research and public health. 2013;10(12):6645-6661.

[30] Mielgo-Ayuso J, Aparicio-Ugarriza R, Castillo A, Ruiz E, Avila JM, Aranceta-Bartrina J, et al. Sedentary behavior among Spanish children and adolescents: findings from the ANIBES study. BMC public health. 2017; 17(1):94.

[31] Carr LJ, Swift M, Ferrer A, Benzo R. Cross-sectional Examination of Long-term Access to Sit-Stand Desks in a Professional Office Setting. American journal of preventive medicine. 2016;50(1):96-100.

[32] O'Donoghue G, Perchoux C, Mensah K, Lakerveld J, van der Ploeg H, Bernaards C, et al. A systematic review of correlates of sedentary behaviour in adults aged 18-65 years: a socio-ecological approach. BMC public health. 2016;16(1):163.

[33] Chastin SF, Buck C, Freiberger E, Murphy M, Brug J, Cardon G, et al. Systematic literature review of determinants of sedentary behaviour in older adults: a DEDIPAC study. The international journal of behavioral nutrition and physical activity. 2015;12:127.

[34] Stierlin AS, De Lepeleere S, Cardon G, Dargent-Molina P, Hoffmann B, Murphy MH, et al. A systematic review of determinants of sedentary behaviour in youth: a DEDIPAC-study. International Journal of Behavioral Nutrition and Physical Activity. 2015;12(1):133.

[35] Brug J, Chinapaw M. Determinants of engaging in sedentary behavior across the lifespan; lessons learned from two systematic reviews conducted within DEDIPAC. International Journal of Behavioral Nutrition and Physical Activity. 2015;12(1):134.

[36] Katzmarzyk PT, Powell KE, Jakicic JM, Troiano RP, Piercy K, Tennant B. Sedentary Behavior and Health: Update from the 2018 Physical Activity Guidelines Advisory Committee. Medicine and science in sports and exercise. 2019;51(6): 1227-1241.

[37] Diaz KM, Howard VJ, Hutto B, Colabianchi N, Vena JE, Safford MM, et al. Patterns of Sedentary Behavior and Mortality in U.S. Middle-Aged and Older Adults. Annals of Internal Medicine. 2017;167(7):465-475.

[38] Boberska M, Szczuka Z, Kruk M, Knoll N, Keller J, Hohl DH, et al. Sedentary behaviours and health-related quality of life. A systematic review and meta-analysis. Health psychology review. 2018;12(2):195-210.

[39] Castro O, Bennie J, Vergeer I, Bosselut G, Biddle SJH. Correlates of sedentary behaviour in university students: A systematic review. Preventive medicine. 2018;116:194-202.

[40] Ramalho A, Petrica J, Rosado A. Sedentary behaviors and psychological outcomes among older adults: a systematic review. Motricidade. 2018;14(1):73-85.

[41] Falck RS, Davis JC, Liu-Ambrose T. What is the association between sedentary behaviour and cognitive function? A systematic review. British journal of sports medicine. 2017;51(10):800-811.

[42] Sui W, Smith ST, Fagan MJ, Rollo S, Prapavessis H. The effects of sedentary behaviour interventions on work-related productivity and performance outcomes in real and simulated office work: A systematic review. Applied ergonomics. 2019;75:27-73.

[43] Zhai L, Zhang Y, Zhang D. Sedentary behaviour and the risk of depression: a meta-analysis. British journal of sports medicine. 2015; 49(11):705.

[44] Teychenne M, Ball K, Salmon J. Sedentary behavior and depression among adults: a review. International journal of behavioral medicine. 2010;17(4):246-254.

[45] Shrestha N, Kukkonen-Harjula KT, Verbeek JH, Ijaz S, Hermans V, Pedisic Z. Workplace interventions for reducing sitting at work. The Cochrane database of systematic reviews. 2018;6(6):Cd010912.

[46] Josaphat K-J, Kugathasan TA, E.R. Reid R, Begon M, Léger P-M, Labonté-Lemoyne E, et al. Use of Active Workstations in Individuals with Overweight or Obesity: A Systematic Review. Obesity. 2019;27(3):362-379.

[47] de Rezende LF, Rey-Lopez JP, Matsudo VK, do Carmo Luiz O. Sedentary behavior and health outcomes among older adults: a systematic review. BMC public health. 2014;14:333.

[48] Wirth K, Klenk J, Brefka S, Dallmeier D, Faehling K, Roqué IFM, et al. Biomarkers associated with sedentary behaviour in older adults: A systematic review. Ageing research reviews. 2017;35:87-111.

[49] Saunders TJ, Atkinson HF, Burr J, MacEwen B, Skeaff CM, Peddie MC. The Acute Metabolic and Vascular Impact of Interrupting Prolonged Sitting: A Systematic Review and Meta-Analysis. Sports medicine (Auckland, NZ). 2018;48(10):2347-66.

[50] Neuhaus M, Eakin EG, Straker L, Owen N, Dunstan DW, Reid N, et al. Reducing occupational sedentary time: a systematic review and meta-analysis of evidence on activity-permissive workstations. Obesity reviews : an official journal of the International Association for the Study of Obesity. 2014;15(10):822-838.

[51] Saunders TJ, McIsaac T, Douillette K, Gaulton N, Hunter S, Rhodes RE, et al. Sedentary behaviour and health in adults: an overview of systematic reviews. Applied physiology, nutrition, and metabolism = Physiologie appliquee, nutrition et metabolisme. 2020;45(10 (Suppl. 2)):S197-s217.

[52] Loh R, Stamatakis E, Folkerts D, Allgrove JE, Moir HJ. Effects of Interrupting Prolonged Sitting with Physical Activity Breaks on Blood Glucose, Insulin and Triacylglycerol Measures: A Systematic Review and Meta-analysis. Sports medicine (Auckland, NZ). 2020;50(2):295-330.

[53] Maylor BD, Zakrzewski-Fruer JK, Stensel DJ, Orton CJ, Bailey DP. Effects of Frequency and Duration of Interrupting Sitting on Cardiometabolic Risk Markers. International journal of sports medicine. 2019;40(13):818-824.

[54] Organization WH. WHO guidelines on physical activity and sedentary behaviour: at a glance. 2020.

[55] Ross R, Chaput JP, Giangregorio LM, Janssen I, Saunders TJ, Kho ME, et al. Canadian 24-Hour Movement Guidelines for Adults aged 18-64 years and Adults aged 65 years or older: an integration of physical activity, sedentary behaviour, and sleep. Applied physiology, nutrition, and metabolism = Physiologie appliquee, nutrition et metabolisme. 2020;45(10 (Suppl. 2)): S57-s102.

[56] Janssen I, Clarke AE, Carson V, Chaput JP, Giangregorio LM, Kho ME, et al. A systematic review of compositional data analysis studies examining associations between sleep, sedentary behaviour, and physical activity with health outcomes in adults. Applied physiology, nutrition, and metabolism = Physiologie appliquee, nutrition et metabolisme. 2020;45(10 (Suppl. 2)):S248-s57.

[57] Ekelund U, Tarp J, Steene-Johannessen J, Hansen BH, Jefferis B,

Fagerland MW, et al. Dose-response associations between accelerometry measured physical activity and sedentary time and all cause mortality: systematic review and harmonised meta-analysis. BMJ. 2019;366:l4570.

[58] Grontved A, Hu FB. Television viewing and risk of type 2 diabetes, cardiovascular disease, and all-cause mortality: a meta-analysis. JAMA. 2011;305(23):2448-2455.

[59] Sun JW, Zhao LG, Yang Y, Ma X, Wang YY, Xiang YB. Association Between Television Viewing Time and All-Cause Mortality: A Meta-Analysis of Cohort Studies. American journal of epidemiology. 2015;182(11):908-916.

[60] Okely AD, Ghersi D, Hesketh KD, Santos R, Loughran SP, Cliff DP, et al. A collaborative approach to adopting/adapting guidelines - The Australian 24-Hour Movement Guidelines for the early years (Birth to 5 years): an integration of physical activity, sedentary behavior, and sleep. BMC public health. 2017;17(Suppl 5):869.

[61] Dutton M. Sit Less, Move More, Sleep Well: Active Play Guidelines for Under-Fives: Ministry of Health; 2017.

[62] Draper CE, Tomaz SA, Biersteker L, Cook CJ, Couper J, de Milander M, et al. The South African 24-Hour Movement Guidelines for Birth to 5 Years: An Integration of Physical Activity, Sitting Behavior, Screen Time, and Sleep. Journal of physical activity & health. 2020;17(1):109-119.

[63] Organization WH. Guidelines on physical activity, sedentary behaviour and sleep for children under 5 years of age: World Health Organization; 2019.

Chapter 2

Methods of Assessing Sedentary Behaviour

Priscila Marconcin, Pedro B. Júdice, Gerson Ferrari, André Werneck and Adilson Marques

Abstract

Increasing amounts of time spent in sedentary behaviour (SB), during occupation or recreation activities, is considered a global health problem. SB has been associated with several non-communicable diseases and all-cause mortality. Thus, it is essential to assess SB through the most accurate and suitable measurement tools. This chapter presents an overview of different methods for assessing SB and highlights the importance of determining the best measurement tool. In choosing an appropriate and accurate method, it is relevant to consider multiple factors, such as population characteristics, context, validity and reliability of measurement tools, and potential research and participant burdens. Subjective measurements, such as self-reported questionnaires, are widely used in epidemiologic studies because they are easy to administer at low cost. However, there is a large variety of questionnaires, which makes it difficult to select a single questionnaire to assess SB. Device-based measurements are more accurate for assessing SB as well as determining bouts and breaks. Both methods present strengths and limitations, and when possible, researchers should use a combination of device-based and subjective methods to improve SB assessment.

Keywords: sitting time, sedentary time, measurement, wearables, self-reported questionnaires

1. Introduction

When James A. Levine[1] said for the first time "sitting is the new smoking," his statement seemed to be dramatic and exaggerated. Still, building evidence contributed to show that he was not entirely wrong. Sedentary behaviour (SB) is systematically associated with numerous health issues, such as prostate cancer [1], breast cancer [2], mental health [3, 4], diabetes, cardiovascular disease [5], and obesity [6]. In addition, SB is associated with all-cause mortality. There is still discussion about whether moderate-to-vigorous physical activity (MVPA) can counteract the

---

[1] James A. Levine is the co-director of the Mayo Clinic/Arizona State University Obesity Solutions Initiative and the inventor of the treadmill desk. He has published more than 100 scientific papers, worked on dozens of corporate programs, and served as an advisor for schools on how to make the classroom a more active place. He is the author of *Get Up!* He won the Invention of the Year Award from NASA, the Platinum Award at the World Fair, and Entrepreneur of the Year in the state of Minnesota. His work has been featured on Rock Center, 60 Minutes, BBC, and all major network US morning shows, as well as in *The New York Times* and *The Times of London*. https://us.macmillan.com/author/jamesalevine/

deleterious effects of SB. However, some investigations show that MVPA and SB are two independent risk factors for mortality rates [7, 8].

The World Health Organisation (WHO) recently updated physical activity (PA) guidelines, considering the minimum amount required to prevent health risks. The recommendations are specific for children, adolescents, adults, and older adults. In addition, subpopulations such as pregnant and postpartum women and people living with chronic conditions or disabilities are included in these new guidelines. For the first time, beyond PA, SB was taken into consideration [9]. Even though SB risk is cited in the PA guidelines, a threshold value is yet to be provided. The WHO points out the importance of periodically reviewing the existing global and national instruments for assessing PA and SB [9]. Therefore, it is essential to accurately measure SB to better understand its role in health outcomes and provide accurate data to update public health guidelines.

SB manifests in different domains (e.g. leisure time, work, transport) and as different types (e.g. working on the computer, watching TV, and playing video games), making it difficult to assess all forms of SB simultaneously. Thus, a clear definition of SB must be provided. In this sense, the Sedentary Behaviour Research Network defined SB as any waking behaviour with energy expenditure ≤1.5 metabolic equivalents (METs) while in a sitting, reclining, or lying posture [10]. **Figure 1** is an interactive figure of the final conceptual model of movement-based terminology arranged around 24 h [10].

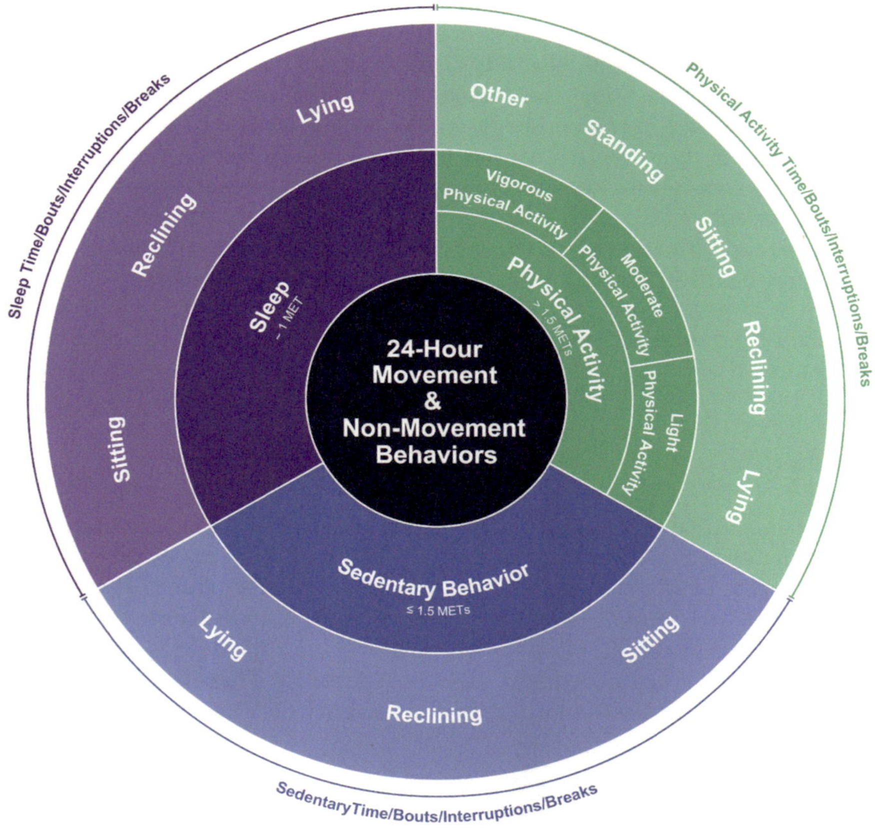

Figure 1.
The conceptual model of movement-based terminology arranged around a 24-h period. The movements are divided into two components. The inner ring represents the main behaviour categories using energy expenditure. The outer ring provides general categories using posture. Source: www.sedentarybehaviour.org/sbrn-terminology-consensus-project/ [10].

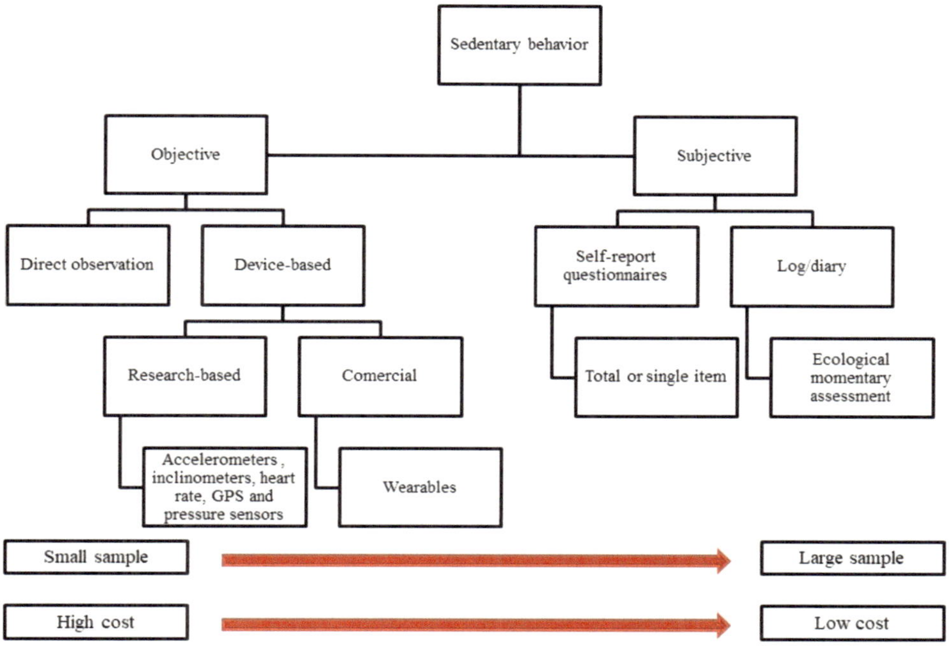

Figure 2.
Flow chart of different methods to assess SB.

Meanwhile, it is quite difficult to adequately assess SB. What parameters of SB should be assessed? Descriptive parameters of SB used frequently are duration, frequency, intensity, and context domains (e.g. leisure, work, transport) [11]. For accurately assessing SB, one must consider not only energy expenditure but also body posture. There is a relatively small absolute difference in energy expenditure between sitting and standing posture, confusing interpretation of the data [12, 13]. Studies show that time spent in continuous prolonged bouts of SB may have the worst health consequence [14–19] and that assessing SB accumulation patterns is paramount.

Device-based measures or subjective methods can assess SB. Both present strengths and limitations that must be considered according to the purpose of the assessment. **Figure 2** summarises the two types of methods and the potential cost and sample size of each. Device-based methods have the greatest validity and are the gold standard for assessing total SB and patterns of SB accumulation. However, these methods alone cannot provide contextual details such as the type of SB, with whom the participant is engaging in the SB, or whether the participant is multi-tasking. Subjective methods, such as self-report questionnaires, give detailed information about the task but are subject to measurement error and response bias. The authors believe that the key to choosing the best assessment approach is to consider the research question and the aim of the study. In this sense, this chapter presents the different methods to assess SB and guides the reader in choosing the appropriate one.

2. Objective methods to assess sedentary behaviour

Table 1 presents an overview of the main objective methods of assessing SB.

Designation	Strengths	Limitations
• To validate novel SB techniques, such as device-based motion sensors • To assess SB in particular sub-population (e.g. Alzheimer's patients)	• Low equipment requirement • Describe with detail the context (activity, posture, breaks in SB) and distinguish the postures (e.g. chair-sitting, ground-sitting, kneeling, and squatting) • High validity and reliability	• Depends on intra- and inter-rater reliability • Quite inconvenient for all those involved • The participant can change their routine, reducing ecological validity • Feasible only with limited sample size, space, and time

Table 1.
Direct observation: designation, strengths, and limitations.

2.1 Direct observation

Direct observation is the gold standard and the most basic method to assess SB. The method consists of two or three trained specialists observing the participant during the timeframe of interest and recording all behaviours and categorising them according to a predetermined list [20]. **Table 2** shows the direct observation details.

2.2 Device-based methods

2.2.1 Methodological considerations

2.2.1.1 Continuously worn devices

Nowadays, it is common for individuals to wear monitoring devices 24 hours per day. Participant compliance is substantially greater with these devices because they do not have to remember to put the device back on after a period of removal. In addition, the risk of bias is reduced when compared to traditionally wearing the devices only while awake. By wearing the devices for 24 h, participants may simply forget that they are using the devices, which can reduce the effect of increasing the usual PA levels.

2.2.1.2 Minimal criteria for having valid data

The protocols are distinct according to the population studied and the device used. For accelerometers, it is common to adopt ≥10 h/day on at least 4 days, including at least one weekend day [22].

2.2.1.3 Acceleration and postural standpoint

It is important to distinguish between "true" SB and other behaviours, such as sleep or non-wear time. To minimise this issue some alternatives are presented: manual evaluations, participant diaries, and automated algorithms.

2.2.1.4 Participants' adherence

It is essential to stimulate the participant to adhere to the assessment. In this sense, it is important to consider the practice to wear and how discreet the device

Characteristics	Accelerometers	Inclinometers	HR monitoring and combined HR and movement monitoring	Multi-sensor monitors
Validity	Medium to high (depending on the processing method)	Very high (≥95% agreement with direct observation)	Low	Low (correlation between activPAL and SenseWear: r = 0.37 (95% CI 0.13, 0.56)
Reliability	Very high	Very high (inter-device reliability >0.99)	Very high	Very high
Participant and research burden	Moderate	Moderate	Participant—low/moderate Researcher—moderate/high	Participant—potentially high Researcher—moderate/high
Cost	Moderate	High	High	High
Strength(s)	A substantial literature on application and analysis.	Able to distinguish sitting/standing, small and discreet underneath clothing, possibility for continuous 24-h wear protocol	Combined movement and physiological data aid the identification of monitor wear time	Able to identify behaviour mode/type
Limitation(s)	No consensus regarding data processing	Validation studies in free-living conditions lacking Adhesive can irritate the wearer's skin	Formal validation studies lacking	Untested in large-scale research settings

Table 2.
Overview of the main device-based methods to assess SB (adapted by Atkin et al. [21] and Aunger and Wagnild [20]).

is. For example, the wrist-worn GENEActiv and Axivity accelerometer devices resemble sport watches, whereas the ActiGraph device is larger and bright red, which may make it less appealing to participants. The activPAL inclinometer is generally inconspicuous on the thigh. Despite common protocols, most of these devices can be positioned in different places, such as on the thigh, potentially increasing the accuracy in measuring SB [23].

2.2.2 Research-based

2.2.2.1 Accelerometers and inclinometers

An accelerometer is a tool that measures the frequency and amplitude of acceleration (counts) of the body in three orthogonal planes (anteroposterior, mediolateral, and vertical) [24]. Time in SB is assessed by two different ways to detect body posture (standing, sitting, or lying): (1) posture by tri-axial sensors using gravitational components or (2) spinal curvature by three uni-axial gyroscopes orthogonally aligned [11]. Alternatively, posture monitors (i.e. inclinometers) seek to distinguish standing, sitting/lying, or sleep/no wear. Considering the definition of SB [10], posture monitors can measure a closer behaviour to SB than accelerometers, and previous studies reported greater agreement for inclinometers with direct observation than accelerometers [25–27]. Although accelerometers are suitable for the fast movement of body segments [28], they are usually used to assess SB in free-living contexts. In addition, they can assess specific segments of the day, such as after school or after work. It is a common method used in epidemiological studies to access PA with the periods of non-movement being interpreted as SB.

Sedentary time has been determined as <100 counts per minute (cpm) on the waist [23] or <1853 cpm on the non-dominant wrist [29].

Accelerometers can be used to detect short breaks in SB. The key issues in the use of accelerometry are the lack of consensus regarding the most appropriate data-processing protocol, limiting comparability between studies and hindering evidence synthesis [21]. For example, the choice of cut-points to distinguish physical behaviours, the allowance or not of momentary interruptions (i.e. seconds) in sedentary bouts, the minimal amount of time to be considered a break in SB, the application of different filters that change the sensitivity of the data, or simply the epoch choice will significantly impact the results and limit comparability among different studies.

There are important considerations regarding the agreement and comparability of SB measurements from accelerometers and inclinometers. Different studies tested the agreement between SB measured through accelerometers and inclinometers and found that accelerometer-based measures of SB can be overestimated, especially in short bouts [30–34]. The overestimation of SB by accelerometers is, in general, low, but this bias can influence the findings of interventions [30]. However, there are potential differences according to placement site. In this sense, a recent investigation examined the agreement between two accelerometers (Actigraph GT3x and Axivity AX3) with the activPAL inclinometer, all placed on the thigh, and found an elevated agreement for sitting time [35].

Accelerometers are generally unobtrusive to wear, quite small, and consume low battery. However, there is reactivity in the use of devices; in other words, the use of a device can change the behaviour, stimulating the practice of PA and/or reducing SB time [36]. In addition, there is an intrinsic error of estimation as accelerometers' estimations (used on the hip or wrist) are based on accelerations and not posture. Consequently, some motionless standing activities can be erroneously classified as SB. Although these devices are very practicable to use in the field, the costs and operationalisation of device-based methods can be a limitation in large population-based studies, especially in middle- and low-income countries.

2.2.2.2 Heart rate monitoring and combined heart rate and movement monitoring

Heart rate (HR) monitoring is the oldest and most recognised method for assessing PA. It estimates the total energy expenditure or time spent at higher PA intensities. HR monitoring uses two different types of technology: the electrical signal (chest belt) and optical sensor (wristwatch or armband) [37]. These sensors are cheap, discrete, and comfortable. The measure is based on the individually calibrated thresholds that differentiate rest from higher-intensity movement (flex-HR method). SB is estimated as daily time spent below the flex-HR threshold.

The relationship between HR and energy expenditure is not linear for the high intensity of PA or at rest and low intensity [38]. Moreover, a similar HR may represent different internal intensities depending on participant age or fitness level, which is another limitation of using HR solely to estimate PA.

The validity of HR to characterise PA intensity is low when low-intensity movement is aimed. This measure of SB generally has high specificity but low sensitivity [21]. Devices that combine HR and accelerometry are available. This makes possible the evaluation of non-movement periods, although in practice these devices have demonstrated poor validity for measuring SB [34].

2.2.2.3 Multi-sensor monitors

Multi-sensor monitors combine accelerometers and physiological sensors (e.g. heat flux, skin temperature). Examples of this type of monitor include the SenseWear Armband and the Intelligent Device for Energy Expenditure and Physical Activity (IDEEA). Their utility in epidemiological domains is unknown, but has been examined in clinical settings [39]. Usually, these devices use multiple sensors attached to various points of the body. The accuracy of these devices was examined in controlled settings, however, the validity and feasibility under free-living conditions have not been extensively tested [21, 40]. These devices are valuable as criterion measures in validating other SB measurement tools but not a good alternative in free-living conditions, as they entail a burden to the participant.

2.2.2.4 Global positioning system (GPS)

The global positioning system (GPS) is the gold-standard, device-based measure to derive location-based data (latitude and longitude) from individuals. It is useful to understand the relationship between varied contexts and active living [41]. In addition, some GPS systems deliver information regarding speed, elevation, and indoor-outdoor activities [11]. However, GPS presents some limitations in assessing indoor activities, especially in tall buildings with small windows. Recent smartphones and smartwatches are equipped with all the mentioned sensors.

2.2.3 Commercial

A wide range of technical specifications is available from wearables. Overall, commercial, wearable devices are small and unobtrusive devices attached and initiated by the users. Acknowledging some differences in the type of sensor embedded in the wearable, the devices usually assess and provide output parameters of general PA and inactivity, energy expenditure, posture, and body movement [42]. The issue with these commercial devices is that the algorithms behind the generated outcomes are never provided to the user, which does not allow a further understanding of how exactly the outcomes are determined.

2.2.3.1 Wearable cameras

These instruments combine device-based measures about the time spent in SB or PA with information about the context and activity. This is especially useful to identify the combined behaviour, for example, watching TV while eating. Although they seem like an ideal method, wearable cameras present ethical/privacy issues that have to do with obtaining consent from third parties to capture images [20].

2.2.3.2 Smartwatches and smartphones

Smartwatches have the potential to help health care by supporting/evaluating health in everyday living. Among other functions, smartwatches can assess SB. Generally, smartwatches tend to underestimate energy expenditure compared to laboratory reference measurements [11]. Due to the ease of access, smartphones are a good alternative to smartwatches or other wearable devices. Currently, smartphones can combine many sensors, such as GPS or Global Navigation Satellite Systems (GLONASS), accelerometers, e-compasses, gyroscopes, proximity sensors, or ambient light sensors [43]. However, the problem is that people not always have their smartphones, so many activities may be missed, which can create bias.

3. Subjective measurements of SB

Table 3 presents an overview of the main subjective methods to assess SB.

3.1 Self-reported questionnaires

Questionnaires are the most popular method to assess SB, but they depend on participant ability to recall. They are mostly used in epidemiologic studies due to their low cost and ease of use, both for researchers and participants. Questionnaires can assess multiple domains of SB, such as duration, frequency, context (e.g. leisure, work, transport), and time of recall (e.g. last week, over the last month). Questionnaires that seek to assess habitual levels of SB are susceptible to random and systematic reporting errors. These tools vary from single-item questions (sometimes asked separately for weekends and weekdays) to extensive questionnaires about SB considering various behaviours or domains. In addition, the assessment can be conducted via different methods, such as on paper, on a computer, or face to face, which impacts the response quality [20].

3.1.1 Single-item questionnaires

Participants should report their SB retrospectively. The most used questionnaire is the International Physical Activity Questionnaire (IPAQ) Short Form, which asks: "During the last 7 days, how much time did you spend sitting on a weekday?" [44] Participants should report the answer in hours and minutes per day. However, this kind of assessment has been demonstrated to underestimate SB. Those questionnaires are subject to social desirability bias or simply reflect the difficulty that participants have in recalling their SB [45, 46]. In large scale, the one-item questionnaire may be preferred, as it showed similar validity and reliability compared to longer questionnaires [47]. If possible, however, researchers must choose multi-item questionnaires to obtain more detailed information, not simply one metric for SB.

3.1.2 Domain-based questionnaires

Domain-based questionnaires ask about specific SB types and estimate total SB by the sum of the time spent in each SB. One example is the Sedentary Behaviour Questionnaire (SBQ), which asks about the time spent in nine SB types (e.g. watching tv, playing games, and seven others) [48]. The composite measure of SB tends to produce more accurate estimates of total SB than single-item recalls. The problem with these questionnaires is they tend to erroneously exceed the SB time when considering multi-tasks. For example, the individual listens to music while using the computer and considers the time of these two activities separately instead of considering a single task (the main one).

The domain-based questionnaires can also ask about specific domains of SB, and in these cases, the validity is usually high [49, 50]. But one must understand that this is a good metric for a single behavior but does not inform about the overall SB.

Characteristics	Total assessment or single-item questionnaires	Domain-based questionnaires (composite)	Domain-based questionnaires (specific behaviour)	Previous-day recall	Diaries	Ecological momentary assessments	Proxy-report methods
Validity	Low (correlation with device-based measures: r = 0.34 (95% CI 0.30, 0.39)	Low for questionnaires with 2–9 items, r = 0.35 (95% CI 0.29, 0.41) compared to device-based measures For questionnaires with ≥10 items r = 0.37 (95% CI 0.30, 0.43) compared to device-based measures	Generally high	High (correlation $\rho > 0.75$ compared to activPAL)	High (correlation r = 0.87)	Low (correlation r = 0.29 compared to activPAL and 0.16 compared to ActiGraph)	Validity largely depends on the validity of the questionnaire being used
Reliability	Variable (intraclass correlations range from 0.41 to 0.86).	Variable (intraclass correlations range from 0.44 to 0.91)	Variable	Medium (lack of evidence, intra-class correlation of 0.75).	Medium (intraclass correlations range from 0.65 to 0.75).	Unknown	Reliability largely depends on the reliability of the questionnaire being used
Participant and researcher burden	Low	Low	Low	Medium	High	High	Low to medium
Cost	Very low	Very low	Very low	Low	Low	Low to high, depending on devices used (e.g., mobile phones)	Very low

Characteristics	Total assessment or single-item questionnaires	Domain-based questionnaires (composite)	Domain-based questionnaires (specific behaviour)	Previous-day recall	Diaries	Ecological momentary assessments	Proxy-report methods
Strength(s)	Easy to administer information on behaviour type and context useful for intervention design.	Easy to administer, provides information on time spent in specific contexts, slightly better estimates of total SB than single-item questionnaires.	Easy to administer	Smaller chance of recall bias Allows inclusion of behaviours relevant to each participant without the imposition of pre-specified behaviours as in a questionnaire	Allows participants to list their activities rather than imposing a structure like in questionnaires Low risk of recall bias if the diary is completed prospectively	Intermittent prompts allow insights into the context of behaviours, including where and with whom they are occurring	Allows measurement of SB in populations who might have difficulty with self-reporting (e.g. adults in need of special care, young children)
Limitation(s)	Typically leads to under-reporting, especially due to difficulty recalling a total sitting time without prompts or possible social desirability bias	Possible recall bias or social desirability bias, concurrent behaviours can lead to double-counting, included behaviours may not be relevant outside of industrialised contexts	Possible recall bias or social desirability bias	More labour-intensive for both participants and researchers compared to questionnaires	Subject to recall and reporting bias, validation studies lacking	Burdensome to participants, prompts can disrupt the actual activity of interest, difficult to gather total SB	Subject to recall and reporting bias, validation studies lacking

Table 3.
Overview of the main subjective methods to assess SB (adapted by Atkin et al. [21] and Aunger and Wagnild [20]).

Another relevant point is that one must use the entire validated questionnaire and not simply use just one question of a valid questionnaire, which will lose validation. Finally, considering that people tend to underestimate SB, and some may not understand the true meaning of the term "sedentary behaviour" due to lack of literacy, these domain-based questionnaires help people to easily identify the time spent in these pursuits, so in this sense they represent an advantage.

3.2 Previous-day recall

Through a semi-structured interview, participants should report in a chronological format the time spent in SB. Activities must last more than 5 minutes to be recorded. Previous-day recall presents a strong correlation ($\rho > 0.75$) with activPAL-measured SB [51, 52]. The biggest limitation of this method is that the previous day may not necessarily be a typical day, thus not representing the typical SB of a participant.

3.3 Diaries and ecological momentary assessments

In diaries, participants must report their daily activities throughout the day. The problem is that if they forget to fill out the questionnaire, they may do it at the end of the day as a retrospective report, which entails more error. The Bouchard Activity Record showed a strong correlation with activPAL-measured SB [53].

Ecological momentary assessment (EMA) is also a prospective record; the difference is that several prompts are sent throughout the day for participants to report their current behaviour. The advantage is that it allows collecting other contextual information, for example, where the participant is carrying out the behaviour and with whom. Both are subject to participants changing their behaviour in response to being monitored. The validity is low, with a weak correlation compared to activPAL [54]. However, EMA showed better correlation and agreement to accelerometer estimates than traditional self-report methods [55].

3.4 Proxy-report methods

Proxy-report methods are useful when participants present some difficulties reporting their behaviours. This occurs with children and adults with cognitive incapacity, so proxy reporting by a third party (usually a parent) can be a good alternative [56]. Proxy-report can be a single-item questionnaire, a diary, or domain-based technique [20]. A systematic review evaluated the reliability and validity of proxy-report methods to assess SB and the results indicate that this measure has acceptable validity (less than 5% of data outside the limits of agreement) [57].

4. Combined device-based and subjective methods

The complexity of SB necessitates more integrated and comprehensive assessment techniques that assess multiple aspects of SB. Device-based methods provide a way to quantify time spent in SB, energy expenditure, position, and other physiological signals but do not inform about contextual features of SB and the type of behaviour that is being partaken. Alternatively, reported methods provide a way to understand the domain, the context, and type of SB. Still, their validity is necessarily lower, as they depend on people's memory and perception. Each method provides unique information, thus neither method alone provides complete information.

In this sense, device-based and subjective methods are potentially complementary, once they capture different aspects of SB. The limitation of one method can be met to some degree by the strength of the other. Whenever feasible, the combination of device-based and subjective assessments will provide the most valid and reliable method to assess SB [47]. The most powerful and useful data collection approach of SB is to integrate the use of reported and device-based methods [56]. For example, HR monitors or accelerometer monitors can be linked wirelessly, with ecological assessment applications on smartphones, and at the same time assess both reported context and perception of SB as well as movement characteristics or physiologic indicators of SB [56] (**Table 4**).

Questionnaire	Summary
Bouchard Physical Activity Questionnaire	A 3-day activity record (including a weekend day). Every 15-min period, participant should report the main activity performed and quantify in terms of energy cost on a 1–9 scale corresponding to a range of 1.0–7.8 METs and higher. Intraclass correlation of 0.96
Previous-Day Recall of Active and Sedentary Behaviours	Participants should report chronologically through the previous day (midnight to midnight) their behaviour using a semi-structured interview. Validation study concluded that: *correlations between the PDR and the activPAL were high, systematic reporting errors were low, and the validity of the PDR was comparable with the ActiGraph.* More information: https://pubmed.ncbi.nlm.nih.gov/23863547/
International Physical Activity Questionnaire (IPAQ)	Participants should report the time spent on different sedentary behaviours. The questionnaire also can be administered over the phone and is available as a short- or long-form and in more than twenty languages/dialects.
Marshall Sitting Questionnaire	A domain-specific sitting questionnaire. Five items assess time (hours and minutes) spent in five different sitting domains. Validation study concluded that: *reliability coefficients were high for a weekday sitting time at work, watching television, and using a computer at home (r = 0.84–0.78) but lower for weekend days across all domains (r = 0.23–0.74). Validity coefficients were highest for weekday sitting at work and using a computer at home (r = 0.69–0.74). With the exception of computer use and watching television for women, the validity of the weekend-day sitting time items was low.* More information: https://pubmed.ncbi.nlm.nih.gov/19997030/
Sedentary Time Questionnaire (SIT-Q)	Asks about the amount of time spent sitting or lying down in different settings over the last 7 days. Validation study concluded that: *ICCs for test–retest reliability ranged from 0.31 for leisure-time computer use to 0.86 for occupational sitting. Total daily sitting demonstrated substantial correlation (ICC = 0.65, 95% CI: 0.49, 0.78).* More information: https://www.sedentarybehaviour.org/wp-content/uploads/2013/12/Lynch-Friedenreich-Khandwala-et-al-2014-2.pdf
The Sedentary Behaviour Questionnaire (SBQ)	Assesses the amount of time spent on nine different behaviours. The validation study concluded that: *ICCs were acceptable for all items and the total scale (range = .51–.93).* More information: https://pubmed.ncbi.nlm.nih.gov/21088299/
The Adolescent Sedentary Activity Questionnaire (ASAQ)	Designed for adolescents. Asks for information regarding different activities: watching television/videos/DVDs, using computers, e-games and e-communication, studying, reading, sitting with friends, using the telephone, listening to or playing music, motorised travel, hobbies and crafts, all performed out of school hours. Validation study concluded that: *test–retest correlations for time total spent in sedentary behaviour were ≥ 0.70, except for Grade 6 boys (Intraclass correlation coefficient (ICC) = 0.57, 95%CI: 0.25, 0.76). Repeatability was generally higher on weekdays compared with weekend days. ICC values for travel and social activities tended to be lower than for the other categories of sedentary behaviour.* More information: https://journals.humankinetics.com/view/journals/jpah/7/6/article-p697.xml

Questionnaire	Summary
Rapid Assessment Disuse Index (RADI)	A questionnaire designed for primary care patients. Validation study concluded that: *RADI was temporally stable (intraclass correlation coefficients 0.79), and a higher score was significantly correlated with greater sedentary time (ρ = 0.40; p < 0.01), fewer sedentary to active transitions (ρ = −0.42; p < 0.01), and less light-intensity physical activity (ρ = −0.40; p < 0.01). The ability of RADI to detect patients with high levels of sedentary time was fair (AUC = 0.72).* More information: https://bjsm.bmj.com/content/48/3/250.abstract
Measure of Older Adults' Sedentary Time (MOST)	A questionnaire designed to assess time spent on behaviours common among older adults. Validation study concluded that: *test–retest reliability was excellent for television viewing time (ρ (95% CI) = 0.78 (0.63–0.89)), computer use (ρ (95% CI) = 0.90 (0.83–0.94)), and reading (ρ (95% CI) = 0.77 (0.62–0.86)); acceptable for hobbies (ρ (95% CI) = 0.61 (0.39–0.76)); and poor for socialising and transport (ρ < 0.45). Total sedentary time had acceptable test–retest reliability (ρ (95% CI) = 0.52 (0.27–0.70)) and validity (ρ (95% CI) = 0.30 (0.02–0.54)). Self-report total sedentary time was similarly responsive to change (RS = 0.47) as accelerometer-derived sedentary time (RS = 0.39).* More information: https://pubmed.ncbi.nlm.nih.gov/21448077/
Past-day Adults' Sedentary Time (PAST)	A seven-item questionnaire about time spent sitting/lying on the previous day for work, transport, television viewing, nonwork computer use, reading, hobbies, and other purposes (summed for total sedentary time). Validation study concluded that: *the PAST had fair to good test–retest reliability (intraclass correlation coefficient = 0.50, 95% confidence interval [CI] = 0.32–0.64). At baseline, the correlation between PAST and activPAL sit/lie time was r = 0.57 (95% CI = 0.39–0.71). The mean difference between PAST at baseline and retest was - 25 min (5.2%), 95% limits of agreement = −5.9 to 5.0 h, and the activPAL sit/lie time was - 9 min (1.8%), 95% limits of agreement = −4.9 to 4.6 h. The PAST showed small but significant responsiveness (−0.44, 95% CI = −0.92 to −0.04); responsiveness of activPAL sit/lie time was not significant.* More information: https://pubmed.ncbi.nlm.nih.gov/23274615/
LASA Sedentary Behaviour Questionnaire	A 10-item questionnaire to assess total sedentary time in older adults. Validation study concluded that: *mean total self-reported sedentary time was 10.4 (SD 3.5) h/d and was not significantly different from mean total device-based sedentary time (10.2 (1.2) h/d, p = 0.63). Total self-reported sedentary time on an average day (sum often activities) correlated moderately (Spearman's r = 0.35, p < 0.01) with total device-based sedentary time. The correlation improved when using the sum of six activities (r = 0.46, p < 0.01), and was much higher than when using TV watching only (r = 0.22, p = 0.05). The test–retest reliability of the sum of six sedentary activities was 0.71 (95% CI 0.57–0.81).* More information: https://bmcgeriatr.biomedcentral.com/track/pdf/10.1186/1471-2318-13-80.pdf
Occupational Sitting and Physical Activity Questionnaire (OSPAQ)	A questionnaire for estimating time spent sitting and standing at work. Validation study concluded that: *the test–retest intraclass correlation coefficients for occupational sitting, standing, and walking for OSPAQ ranged from 0.73 to 0.90, while that for the modified MOSPA-Q [a separate questionnaire] ranged from 0.54 to 0.89. Comparison of sitting measures with accelerometers showed higher Spearman correlations for the OSPAQ (r = 0.65) than for the modified MOSPA-Q (r = 0.52). Criterion validity correlations for occupational standing and walking measures were comparable for both instruments with accelerometers (standing:r = 0.49; walking:r = 0.27–0.29).* More information: https://pubmed.ncbi.nlm.nih.gov/21659903/
NIGHTLY-WEEK-U (adapted from the Past-day Adults' Sedentary Time-University (PAST-U))	Adapted from the Past-day Adults' Sedentary Time-University (PAST-U): the PAST-WEEK-U and the NIGHTLY-WEEK-U. Validation study concluded that: *the average sedentary time (ST) captured using the NIGHTLY-WEEK-U was 0.21 h lower than the criterion measure activPAL4™ (i.e., 10.50 vs 10.29 h per day), with a 95% limit of agreement ranging from −1.75 to 2.17 h. The NIGHTLY-WEEK-U provides a superior measure of ST compared with the PAST-WEEK-U and potentially other weekly measures of ST.* More information: https://onlinelibrary.wiley.com/doi/full/10.1002/tsm2.123

Available: /www.sedentarybehaviour.org/sedentary-behaviour-questionnaires/).

Table 4.
Validated questionnaires for sedentary behaviour (based on sedentary behaviour research network).

5. Conclusion

Accurate methods to assess SB are essential to promote a more comprehensive advantage in the epidemiological field. In this chapter, we described the various methods of measuring SB and highlighted their limitations and strengths. Assessment of SB by subjective methods is limited by the ubiquitous nature of the SB and therefore difficult to recall. However, questionnaires are the most practical and economical means for large samples. Alternatively, device-based measurements extinguish the possibility of recall bias or subjective overestimation/underestimation depending on the population group and even acknowledging some limitations. They provide more accurate and reliable information on posture, movement (or lack of movement), and accumulation patterns.

To select the most suitable method to assess SB and correctly interpret the measures obtained, researchers must consider the aim of assessment, SB constructs of interest, time factors, and the characteristics and size of the population to be investigated.

Conflict of interest

The authors declare no conflict of interest.

Author details

Priscila Marconcin[1], Pedro B. Júdice[2], Gerson Ferrari[3], André Werneck[4] and Adilson Marques[1*]

1 Faculty of Human Kinetics, Lisbon, Portugal

2 CIDEFES, Univerdade Lusófona de Humanidades e Tecnologias, Lisbon, Portugal

3 Universidad de Santiago de Chile, Santiago, Chile

4 University of São Paulo, São Paulo, Brazil

*Address all correspondence to: adncmpt@gmail.com

References

[1] Berger FF, Leitzmann MF, Hillreiner A, Sedlmeier AM, Prokopidi-Danisch ME, Burger M, et al. Sedentary behavior and prostate cancer: A systematic review and meta-analysis of prospective Cohort studies. Cancer Prevention Research (Philadelphia, Pa). 2019;**12**(10):675-688. DOI: 10.1158/1940-6207.capr-19-0271

[2] Chan DSM, Abar L, Cariolou M, Nanu N, Greenwood DC, Bandera EV, et al. World cancer research fund international: Continuous update project-systematic literature review and meta-analysis of observational cohort studies on physical activity, sedentary behavior, adiposity, and weight change and breast cancer risk. Cancer Causes & Control: CCC. 2019;**30**(11):1183-1200. DOI: 10.1007/s10552-019-01223-w

[3] Stanczykiewicz B, Banik A, Knoll N, Keller J, Hohl DH, Rosińczuk J, et al. Sedentary behaviors and anxiety among children, adolescents and adults: A systematic review and meta-analysis. BMC Public Health. 2019;**19**(1):459. DOI: 10.1186/s12889-019-6715-3

[4] Suchert V, Hanewinkel R, Isensee B. Sedentary behavior and indicators of mental health in school-aged children and adolescents: A systematic review. Preventive Medicine. 2015;**76**:48-57. DOI: 10.1016/j.ypmed.2015.03.026

[5] Wilmot EG, Edwardson CL, Achana FA, Davies MJ, Gorely T, Gray LJ, et al. Sedentary time in adults and the association with diabetes, cardiovascular disease and death: Systematic review and meta-analysis. Diabetologia. 2012;**55**(11):2895-2905. DOI: 10.1007/s00125-012-2677-z

[6] Azevedo LB, Ling J, Soos I, Robalino S, Ells L. The effectiveness of sedentary behaviour interventions for reducing body mass index in children and adolescents: Systematic review and meta-analysis. Obesity Reviews: An Official Journal of the International Association for the Study of Obesity. 2016;**17**(7):623-635. DOI: 10.1111/obr.12414

[7] Diaz KM, Howard VJ, Hutto B, Colabianchi N, Vena JE, Safford MM, et al. Patterns of sedentary behavior and mortality in U.S. middle-aged and older adults. Annals of Internal Medicine. 2017;**167**(7):465-475. DOI: 10.7326/M17-0212

[8] Young Deborah R, Hivert M-F, Alhassan S, Camhi Sarah M, Ferguson Jane F, Katzmarzyk Peter T, et al. Sedentary behavior and cardiovascular morbidity and mortality: A science advisory from the American Heart Association. Circulation. 2016;**134**(13):e262-ee79. DOI: 10.1161/CIR.0000000000000440

[9] WHO. WHO Guidelines on Physical Activity and Sedentary Behaviour: at a Glance. 2020. Geneva: World Health Organization.

[10] Tremblay MS, Aubert S, Barnes JD, Saunders TJ, Carson V, Latimer-Cheung AE, et al. Sedentary Behavior Research Network (SBRN)—Terminology consensus project process and outcome. International Journal of Behavioral Nutrition and Physical Activity. 2017;**14**(1):75. DOI: 10.1186/s12966-017-0525-8

[11] Boudet G, Chausse P, Thivel D, Rousset S, Mermillod M, Baker JS, et al. How to measure sedentary behavior at work? Frontiers in Public Health. 2019;7:167. DOI: 10.3389/fpubh.2019.00167

[12] Gibbs BB, Kowalsky RJ, Perdomo SJ, Grier M, Jakicic JM. Energy expenditure of deskwork when sitting, standing or alternating positions. Occupational

Medicine (Oxford, England). 2017;**67**(2):121-127. DOI: 10.1093/occmed/kqw115

[13] Júdice PB, Hamilton MT, Sardinha LB, Zderic TW, Silva AM. What is the metabolic and energy cost of sitting, standing and sit/stand transitions? European Journal of Applied Physiology. 2016;**116**(2):263-273. DOI: 10.1007/s00421-015-3279-5

[14] Segura-Jiménez V, Gavilán-Carrera B, Acosta-Manzano P, Cook DB, Estévez-López F, Delgado-Fernández M. Sedentary time accumulated in bouts is positively associated with disease severity in fibromyalgia: The Al-Ándalus project. Journal of Clinical Medicine. 2020;**9**(3):733. DOI: 10.3390/jcm9030733

[15] Peddie MC, Bone JL, Rehrer NJ, Skeaff CM, Gray AR, Perry TL. Breaking prolonged sitting reduces postprandial glycemia in healthy, normal-weight adults: A randomized crossover trial. The American Journal of Clinical Nutrition. 2013;**98**(2):358-366. DOI: 10.3945/ajcn.112.051763

[16] Ellingson LD, Meyer JD, Shook RP, Dixon PM, Hand GA, Wirth MD, et al. Changes in sedentary time are associated with changes in mental wellbeing over 1 year in young adults. Preventive Medicine Reports. 2018;**11**:274-281. DOI: 10.1016/j.pmedr.2018.07.013

[17] Healy GN, Dunstan DW, Salmon J, Cerin E, Shaw JE, Zimmet PZ, et al. Breaks in sedentary time: Beneficial associations with metabolic risk. Diabetes Care. 2008;**31**(4):661-666. DOI: 10.2337/dc07-2046

[18] Júdice PB, Silva AM, Berria J, Petroski EL, Ekelund U, Sardinha LB. Sedentary patterns, physical activity and health-related physical fitness in youth: A cross-sectional study. The International Journal of Behavioral Nutrition and Physical Activity. 2017;**14**(1):25. DOI: 10.1186/s12966-017-0481-3

[19] Santos DA, Magalhães JP, Júdice PB, Correia IR, Minderico CS, Ekelund U, et al. Fitness mediates activity and sedentary patterns associations with adiposity in youth. Medicine and Science in Sports and Exercise. 2019;**51**(2):323-329. DOI: 10.1249/mss.0000000000001785

[20] Aunger J, Wagnild J. Objective and subjective measurement of sedentary behavior in human adults: A toolkit. American Journal of Human Biology. 2020;**n/a**(n/a):e23546. DOI: 10.1002/ajhb.23546

[21] Atkin AJ, Gorely T, Clemes SA, Yates T, Edwardson C, Brage S, et al. Methods of measurement in epidemiology: Sedentary behaviour. International Journal of Epidemiology. 2012;**41**(5):1460-1471. DOI: 10.1093/ije/dys118

[22] Healy GN, Clark BK, Winkler EA, Gardiner PA, Brown WJ, Matthews CE. Measurement of adults' sedentary time in population-based studies. American Journal of Preventive Medicine. 2011;**41**(2):216-227. DOI: 10.1016/j.amepre.2011.05.005

[23] Matthews CE, Chen KY, Freedson PS, Buchowski MS, Beech BM, Pate RR, et al. Amount of time spent in sedentary behaviors in the United States, 2003-2004. American Journal of Epidemiology. 2008;**167**(7):875-881. DOI: 10.1093/aje/kwm390

[24] Chen KY, Bassett DR Jr. The technology of accelerometry-based activity monitors: Current and future. Medicine and Science in Sports and Exercise. 2005;**37**(11 Suppl):S490-S500. DOI: 10.1249/01.mss.0000185571.49104.82

[25] Bassett DR, John D, Conger SA, Rider BC, Passmore RM, Clark JM.

Detection of lying down, sitting, standing, and stepping using two activPAL monitors. Medicine and Science in Sports and Exercise. 2014;**46**(10):2025-2029. DOI: 10.1249/mss.0000000000000326

[26] Chinapaw MJM, de Niet M, Verloigne M, De Bourdeaudhuij I, Brug J, Altenburg TM. From sedentary time to sedentary patterns: Accelerometer data reduction decisions in youth. PloS One. 2014;**9**(11):e111205-e. DOI: 10.1371/journal.pone.0111205

[27] Keadle SK, Shiroma EJ, Freedson PS, Lee IM. Impact of accelerometer data processing decisions on the sample size, wear time and physical activity level of a large cohort study. BMC Public Health. 2014;**14**:1210. DOI: 10.1186/1471-2458-14-1210

[28] Plamondon A, Delisle A, Larue C, Brouillette D, McFadden D, Desjardins P, et al. Evaluation of a hybrid system for three-dimensional measurement of trunk posture in motion. Applied Ergonomics. 2007;**38**(6):697-712. DOI: 10.1016/j.apergo.2006.12.006

[29] Koster A, Shiroma EJ, Caserotti P, Matthews CE, Chen KY, Glynn NW, et al. Comparison of sedentary estimates between activPAL and Hip- and Wrist-Worn ActiGraph. Medicine and Science in Sports and Exercise. 2016;**48**(8):1514-1522. DOI: 10.1249/mss.0000000000000924

[30] Silva DR, Minderico CS, Júdice PB, Werneck AO, Ohara D, Cyrino ES, et al. Agreement between GT3X accelerometer and ActivPAL inclinometer for estimating and detecting changes in different contexts of sedentary time among adolescents. Journal of Physical Activity & Health. 2019;**16**(9):780-784. DOI: 10.1123/jpah.2018-0178

[31] De Decker E, De Craemer M, Santos-Lozano A, Van Cauwenberghe E, De Bourdeaudhuij I, Cardon G. Validity of the ActivPAL™ and the ActiGraph monitors in preschoolers. Medicine and Science in Sports and Exercise. 2013;**45**(10):2002-2011. DOI: 10.1249/MSS.0b013e318292c575

[32] Carlson JA, Bellettiere J, Kerr J, Salmon J, Timperio A, Verswijveren S, et al. Day-level sedentary pattern estimates derived from hip-worn accelerometer cut-points in 8-12-year-olds: Do they reflect postural transitions? Journal of Sports Sciences. 2019;**37**(16):1899-1909. DOI: 10.1080/02640414.2019.1605646

[33] Júdice PB, Teixeira L, Silva AM, Sardinha LB. Accuracy of Actigraph inclinometer to classify free-living postures and motion in adults with overweight and obesity. Journal of Sports Sciences. 2019;**37**(15):1708-1716. DOI: 10.1080/02640414.2019.1586281

[34] Júdice PB, Santos DA, Hamilton MT, Sardinha LB, Silva AM. Validity of GT3X and Actiheart to estimate sedentary time and breaks using ActivPAL as the reference in free-living conditions. Gait & Posture. 2015;**41**(4):917-922. DOI: 10.1016/j.gaitpost.2015.03.326

[35] Crowley P, Skotte J, Stamatakis E, Hamer M, Aadahl M, Stevens ML, et al. Comparison of physical behavior estimates from three different thigh-worn accelerometers brands: A proof-of-concept for the Prospective Physical Activity, Sitting, and Sleep consortium (ProPASS). The International Journal of Behavioral Nutrition and Physical Activity. 2019;**16**(1):65. DOI: 10.1186/s12966-019-0835-0

[36] Davis RE, Loprinzi PD. Examination of accelerometer reactivity among a population sample of children, adolescents, and adults. Journal of Physical Activity & Health. 2016;**13**(12):1325-1332. DOI: 10.1123/jpah.2015-0703

[37] Shelley KH. Photoplethysmography: Beyond the calculation of arterial oxygen saturation and heart rate. Anesthesia and Analgesia. 2007;**105**(6 Suppl):S31-S36, tables of contents. DOI: 10.1213/01.ane.0000269512.82836.c9

[38] Livingstone MB. Heart-rate monitoring: The answer for assessing energy expenditure and physical activity in population studies? The British Journal of Nutrition. 1997;**78**(6):869-871. DOI: 10.1079/bjn19970205

[39] Culhane KM, O'Connor M, Lyons D, Lyons GM. Accelerometers in rehabilitation medicine for older adults. Age Ageing. 2005;**34**(6):556-560. DOI: 10.1093/ageing/afi192

[40] Sardinha LB, Júdice PB. Usefulness of motion sensors to estimate energy expenditure in children and adults: A narrative review of studies using DLW. European Journal of Clinical Nutrition. 2017;**71**(8):1026. DOI: 10.1038/ejcn.2017.78

[41] Katapally TR, Bhawra J, Patel P. A systematic review of the evolution of GPS use in active living research: A state of the evidence for research, policy, and practice. Health & Place. 2020;**66**:102453. DOI: https://doi.org/10.1016/j.healthplace.2020.102453

[42] Holtermann A, Schellewald V, Mathiassen SE, Gupta N, Pinder A, Punakallio A, et al. A practical guidance for assessments of sedentary behavior at work: A PEROSH initiative. Applied Ergonomics. 2017;**63**:41-52. DOI: 10.1016/j.apergo.2017.03.012

[43] Reeder B, David A. Health at hand: A systematic review of smart watch uses for health and wellness. Journal of Biomedical Informatics. 2016;**63**:269-276. DOI: https://doi.org/10.1016/j.jbi.2016.09.001

[44] Craig CL, Marshall AL, Sjöström M, Bauman AE, Booth ML, Ainsworth BE, et al. International physical activity questionnaire: 12-country reliability and validity. Medicine and Science in Sports and Exercise. 2003;**35**(8):1381-1395. DOI: 10.1249/01.mss.0000078924.61453.fb

[45] Jefferis BJ, Sartini C, Ash S, Lennon LT, Wannamethee SG, Whincup PH. Validity of questionnaire-based assessment of sedentary behaviour and physical activity in a population-based cohort of older men; comparisons with objectively measured physical activity data. International Journal of Behavioral Nutrition and Physical Activity. 2016;**13**(1):1-11

[46] Van Cauwenberg J, Van Holle V, De Bourdeaudhuij I, Owen N, Deforche B. Older adults' reporting of specific sedentary behaviors: Validity and reliability. BMC Public Health. 2014;**14**(1):734. DOI: 10.1186/1471-2458-14-734

[47] Bakker EA, Hartman YAW, Hopman MTE, Hopkins ND, Graves LEF, Dunstan DW, et al. Validity and reliability of subjective methods to assess sedentary behaviour in adults: A systematic review and meta-analysis. International Journal of Behavioral Nutrition and Physical Activity. 2020;**17**(1):75. DOI: 10.1186/s12966-020-00972-1

[48] Rosenberg DE, Norman GJ, Wagner N, Patrick K, Calfas KJ, Sallis JF. Reliability and validity of the Sedentary Behavior Questionnaire (SBQ) for adults. Journal of Physical Activity & Health. 2010;**7**(6):697-705. DOI: 10.1123/jpah.7.6.697

[49] Grøntved A, Hu FB. Television viewing and risk of type 2 diabetes, cardiovascular disease, and all-cause mortality: A meta-analysis. Jama. 2011;**305**(23):2448-2455. DOI: 10.1001/jama.2011.812

[50] van Uffelen JG, Wong J, Chau JY, van der Ploeg HP, Riphagen I,

Gilson ND, et al. Occupational sitting and health risks: A systematic review. American Journal of Preventive Medicine. 2010;**39**(4):379-388. DOI: 10.1016/j.amepre.2010.05.024

[51] Gomersall SR, Pavey TG, Clark BK, Jasman A, Brown WJ. Validity of a self-report recall tool for estimating sedentary behavior in adults. Journal of Physical Activity & Health. 2015;**12**(11):1485-1491. DOI: 10.1123/jpah.2014-0602

[52] Matthews CE, Keadle SK, Sampson J, Lyden K, Bowles HR, Moore SC, et al. Validation of a previous-day recall measure of active and sedentary behaviors. Medicine and Science in Sports and Exercise. 2013;**45**(8):1629-1638. DOI: 10.1249/MSS.0b013e3182897690

[53] Hart TL, McClain JJ, Tudor-Locke C. Controlled and free-living evaluation of objective measures of sedentary and active behaviors. Journal of Physical Activity & Health. 2011;**8**(6):848-857. DOI: 10.1123/jpah.8.6.848

[54] Maher JP, Rebar AL, Dunton GF. Ecological momentary assessment is a feasible and valid methodological tool to measure older adults' physical activity and sedentary behavior. Frontiers in Psychology. 2018;**9**:1485. DOI: 10.3389/fpsyg.2018.01485

[55] Knell G, Gabriel KP, Businelle MS, Shuval K, Wetter DW, Kendzor DE. Ecological momentary assessment of physical activity: Validation study. Journal of Medical Internet Research. 2017;**19**(7):e253-e. DOI: 10.2196/jmir.7602

[56] Richard PT, Kelley KPG, Gregory JW, Neville O, Barbara S. Reported physical activity and sedentary behavior: Why do you ask? Journal of Physical Activity and Health. 2012;**9**(s1):S68-S75. DOI: 10.1123/jpah.9.s1.s68

[57] Lubans DR, Hesketh K, Cliff DP, Barnett LM, Salmon J, Dollman J, et al. A systematic review of the validity and reliability of sedentary behaviour measures used with children and adolescents. Obesity Reviews : An Official Journal of the International Association for the Study of Obesity. 2011;**12**(10):781-799. DOI: 10.1111/j.1467-789X.2011.00896.x

Chapter 3

The Application of EMG-Based Methods in Evaluating the Impact of Prolonged Sitting on People's Health

Bochen Jia

Abstract

This chapter demonstrates a practical application of electromyography (EMG) technology in assessing the potential negative impacts of new trends (i.e., prolonged sitting) in life and work on people's health. With the development of advanced technologies, prolonged sitting, have become more frequent at work and in everyday life. The potential risks associated with prolonged sitting can be assessed by evaluating localized muscle states using various EMG-based methods. However, due to the unique characteristics of prolonged sitting (i.e., sustained low-load condition), there are several challenges in applying traditional EMG methods to estimate the prolonged sitting related risks. Therefore, from the following aspects, this chapter discusses the potential applications and challenges of using surface EMG-based methods in identifying the effects of prolonged sitting: (1) what are the unique characteristics of the task conditions involved in prolonged sitting; (2) what are the available EMG-based methods; and (3) the advantage and disadvantage of each method in evaluating the impacts of prolonged sitting on people's health;

Keywords: muscle fatigue, prolonged sitting, low Back pain, EMG, muscle stimulation

1. Introduction

Electromyography (EMG) is an electrodiagnostic technique for assessing the contractile activity produced by skeletal muscles. Through electrodes placed on top of the skin's surface, surface EMG signals can detect neuromuscular states and abnormalities, muscle contraction levels, muscle recruitment order, and disorders of motor control and can estimate muscle forces and human movement.

By understanding the muscle state via EMG, the impacts of modern lifestyles and work conditions on the human musculoskeletal system that could lead to potential injuries and illnesses, such as low back pain (LBP), may be identified. LBP is one of the most common societal health problems, causing day away from works, high health services cost, and considerable disability. LBP is one of the leading factors that cause injuries and disability among those under 43 years old [1]. More than 38% of work-related musculoskeletal disorders can be linked to back disorders each year, with a total of 134,550 cases reported in the United States in 2016 [1].

As a new trend in both modern living and contemporary work, sedentary behaviors have become more and more prevalent. Prolonged sitting as a form of sedentary behavior presents emerging health risks in both occupational and non-occupational settings [2]. Sitting is commonly considered a critical ergonomic exposure related to LBP [3, 4]. Recent research has found that muscle activation levels around the lumbar area increase over time during sitting [5, 6] and cause higher levels of muscle co-contractions [7], which have been shown to positively correlate to the development of low back pain [6, 7].

During the sitting, postural muscles, such as trunk extensors, are required to stabilize the sitting posture via sustained contractions, which, however, usually require very low levels of muscle contractions (<10% of maximal muscle capacity) [8, 9]. However, after a long exposure duration, seated posture could block muscle oxygenation and blood flow [10], cause lumbar muscle fatigue, increase intradiscal loads, and further contribute to the development of LBP [11, 12]. Therefore, even though the muscle contraction level during sitting is low, the sustained contractions may cause above mentioned issues even after a continuous duration only greater than 20 minutes [13, 14]. After a long period of sitting (i.e., >90 min), EMG median power frequency has also been observed to shift to the lower frequencies [15, 16]. Even though there is evidence that EMG can measure muscle fatigue caused by sitting, it is generally believed that 15% of muscle contraction level (compared to maximum muscle contraction capacity) is required to detect and distinguish fatigue-induced EMG changes from noises [21]. Both lowered EMG median frequency and increased EMG amplitudes under consistent workloads are generally considered a sign of muscle fatigue [15]. However, such methods may lead to conflicting results when detecting muscle fatigue under low-level contractions.

Therefore, EMG-related measurements provide potential paths to reveal the underneath mechanisms that link prolonged sitting with LBP. At the same time, some potential challenges may affect measurement performance. Therefore, in this chapter, using a prolonged sitting experiment as an example, a series of EMG-based muscle fatigue measurement methods are discussed with respect to their capabilities and limitations in quantifying the negative impacts of prolonged sitting.

2. Determining the effects of prolonged sitting using EMG-based muscle fatigue measurement methods

2.1 Study design

Six participants [gender balanced, mean age (SD) = 25.1 (3.3) yrs] were recruited from the local community to complete a one-hour prolonged seated task. As shown in **Figure 1**, participants were required to sit in a relaxed posture without significant in-chair body movements, such as trunk rotation or bending that could cause significant off-sagittal plane movement. No use of backrest was allowed to minimize potential confounding effects caused by the backrest support on muscle activation pattern during the experiment.

During the experiments, participants were asked to conduct a relaxed internet browsing task to minimize the potential impacts of high mental workloads on muscle activities. The browsing tasks were self-selected with a similar level of mental/physical workloads, e.g., participants can choose to browse websites or stream videos but cannot play intense games or other high demanding tasks. All participants read and signed an informed consent with IRB approval prior to participation.

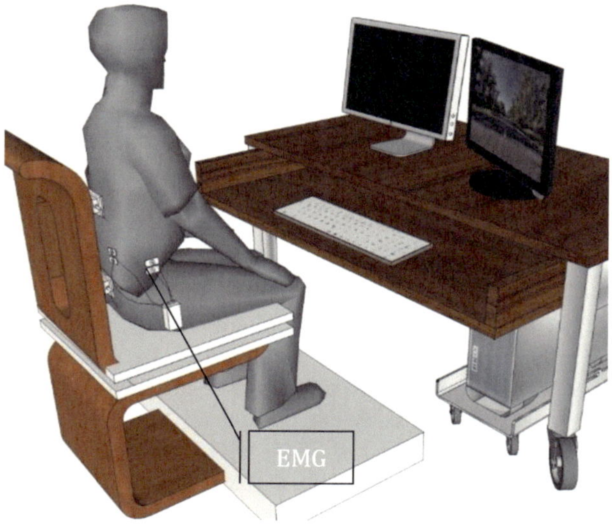

Figure 1.
Illustration of seating device and seated tasks.

2.2 EMG data collection and analysis

To understand how muscles support the trunk against the continuous sitting, the major muscles around the lumbar spine should be studied. In detail, sixteen muscles around the lower lumbar region were studied, which can usually be categorized into the trunk flexors group and the trunk extensors group based on the different function of each muscle. Trunk flexors are those dominant muscles that drive trunk flexion movement, while trunk extensors are those dominant muscles that lead the trunk extension movement. Trunk sideways bending and rotation usually are the results of the combined muscle activities from trunk flexors and extensors.

The tested trunk flexors group includes internal oblique (IO), external oblique (EO), and rectus abdominis (RA). The tested trunk extensors group includes iliocostalis lumborum pars lumborum (ILL), iliocostalis lumborum pars thoracis (ILT), multifidus (MF), longissimus thoracis pars lumborum (LTL), and longissimus thoracis pars thoracis (LTT). Both trunk flexors and extensors can be further divided bilaterally into the left side (L) and the right side (R). The deeper trunk muscles (e.g., psoas, quadratus lumborum, and transverse abdominis) are not included in the analysis due to the fact that such deeper muscles cannot be measured through surface EMG and do not significantly contribute to lumbar kinetics [17]. Each muscle is composed of a group of functional fascicles, each of which has distinct insertion, via, and origin points attached to the bone, which represent the diverse anatomy within each muscle. The initial insertion, via, and origin points are defined as the attach or wrap points where the muscles connect to the bone [18]. For these sixteen trunk muscles, there are a total of ninety-two fascicles (EO = 4, IO = 12, RA = 4, MF = 24, ILL = 8, ILT = 16, LTL = 10, LTT = 14). Equal contraction level is usually assumed among all the fascicles from the same muscle [19]. During trunk movement, each fascicle moves differently due to the different insertion, via, and origin points positions on the bone. Measured trunk kinematics can be used to estimate the line of action and length of each fascicle at each sample instant. So, the EMG activity measured from surface EMG devices can be used to describe the muscle contraction levels.

To monitor and collect muscle EMG data over a long period, a high-fidelity multimodal EMG system is required to collect reliable data continuously with flexible measurement options. A wireless EMG system (Trigno™, Delsys, MA) is included in this chapter. The Trigno wireless EMG system supports up to 16 wireless sensors, which can be used to monitor all 16 muscles simultaneously. To maximize the quality of the collected data, skin near the central position over the muscle belly (but not directly over motor points) of each target muscle was shaved, abrased, and cleaned with a mild alcohol solution to ensure that the impedance was lower than 10 KΩ. Electrodes were placed bilaterally over the surface of each muscle, as suggested in [20]. Raw EMG single amplitude usually ranges from −5000 to 5000 microvolts with frequency ranges between 10 and 500 Hz, in which most frequency power lies between 20 and 400 Hz. Using the Trigno system, raw EMG signals were collected at 2000 Hz, pre-amplified at 500 gain, and band-pass filtered between 20 and 400 Hz. To further smooth the signal, the root-mean-square (RMS) of EMG was calculated using a 200-milliseconds sliding window for the relatively static task, i.e., sitting. Then RMS EMG of the same muscle collected bilaterally were averaged since no significant off-sagittal plane in-chair movements were allowed during the experiment. Collected EMG data were furthered analyzed to answer the following questions for a better understanding of the impact of the prolonged sitting:

The first question is how much effort the related muscles have to contribute continuously to maintaining a seated posture for a prolonged duration. By answering this question, the neuromuscular demands required during prolonged seated tasks could be determined, and a corresponding ergonomics intervention can be developed to lower the stress and strain on workers.

To answer this question, the muscles' contraction levels relative to their maximum capacity need to be determined. Muscle EMG collected from a maximum voluntary contraction (MVC) test can be used as a reference of 100% muscle capacity, and muscle EMG measured during a task can be normalized to this reference to generate the percentage of effort needed to complete the task. The MVC values of all sixteen muscles were measured from suggested MVC tests [20, 21]. Once the MVC value for each muscle is determined, the muscle EMG during prolonged sitting can be converted into the percentage of the MVC value to estimate the level of neuromuscular effort needed for the prolonged sitting [22].

As shown in **Figure 2**, the average muscle activation levels over the entire one hour sitting are generally less than 10% MVC. However, unlike other physically demanding tasks, the exposure duration in such low load seated tasks is long, necessitating a significant amount of time for the muscles to recover from previous fatigue [11].

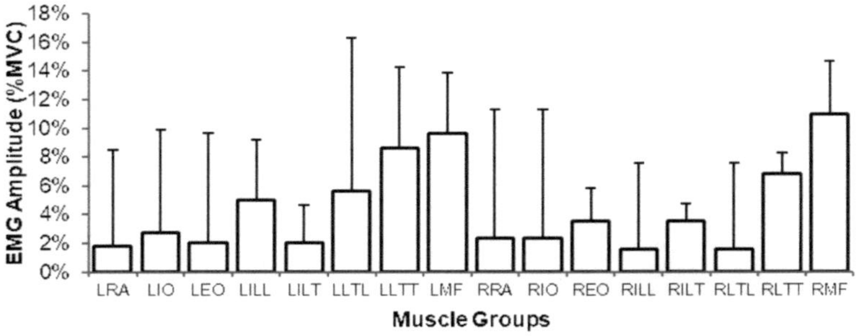

Figure 2.
Average muscle contraction level (%MVC) over the prolonged seated task.

The second question is whether there is any muscle fatigue developed during prolonged sitting. Muscle fatigue is one of the leading indicators that directly link to the development of LBP. Traditionally, both EMG amplitude and EMG median frequency show time-domain changes due to muscular fatigue. Therefore, monitoring EMG amplitude changes over time during prolonged sitting can estimate the level of muscle fatigue development. Using EMG amplitude, muscle fatigue is defined as an amplitude increase over time without an increase in the level of physical demands.

In this study, EMG amplitudes were continuously collected for one minute, and this procedure was repeated every ten minutes. The collected EMG over one minute was then averaged to present the general trend at each data collection period during prolonged sitting. As shown in **Figure 3**, EMG amplitude collected from both muscle groups, in general, increased toward the end of the sitting period. Both LMF and LLTT have a significant increase in measured EMG amplitude. Such an upward change trend, however, was not consistent and fluctuated up and down, which could further indicate that many moderating factors, such as body movement and external forces, could have affected the amplitudes of the collected muscle EMG.

The second indicator is the median power frequency (MPF) of raw EMG obtained from the prolonged sitting. Such MPF was calculated over 3-second windows. As described above, EMG data were continuously collected for one minute every ten minutes, and the mean EMG MPF from each one-minute period was calculated and compared. Changes between these mean values were used as a predictor of fatigue development in these muscles. Multivariate analysis of variance (MANOVA, using Wilks' Lambda) was used to determine the effects of prolonged sitting on all EMG MPFs as a whole. In the event of a significant MANOVA effect, univariate ANOVAs were performed to determine which muscle was mostly impacted by the prolonged seated task, which was considered significant when $p < 0.05$.

MANOVA results indicated that prolonged sitting ($p < 0.01$) had significant effects on the tested EMG MPFs. As shown in **Table 1**, subsequent univariate ANOVAs indicated that prolonged sitting significantly affected MPFs from some of the muscles, which manifested as a declining percentage of EMG MPF: left side LILL (16%) and LLTT (18%) muscles and right side RMF (14%) and RIO (8%) muscles.

As mentioned above, muscle contraction at 15% MVC or higher is usually considered to be the minimal muscle contraction level to detect fatigue-related

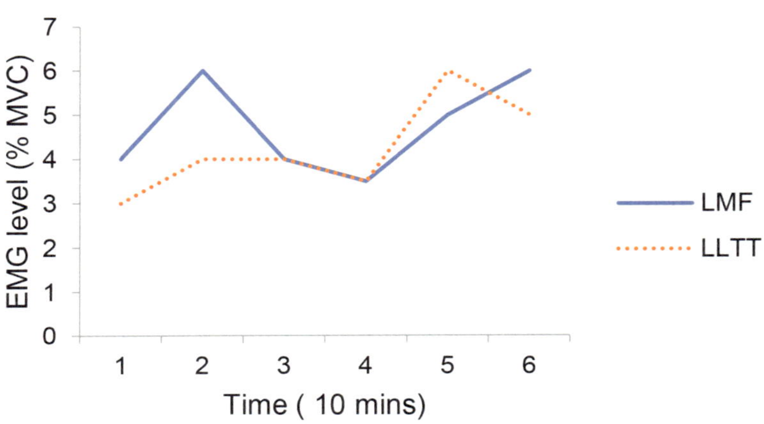

Figure 3.
An example of EMG amplitude (LMF and LLTT) changes over the one-hour prolonged seated task.

		Prolonged Sitting	
		$F_{(1,320)}$	p
EMG Median Frequency	LMF	2.16	0.15
	LILL	7.65	**<0.01**
	LILT	3.36	0.06
	LLTL	3.37	0.88
	LLTT	9.16	**<0.01**
	LEO	3.46	0.06
	LIO	4.51	0.05
	LRA	2.71	0.12
	RMF	5.58	**0.02**
	RILL	4.25	0.06
	RILT	4.34	0.06
	RLTL	3.17	0.08
	RLTT	4.02	0.06
	REO	0.03	0.86
	RIO	4.98	**0.04**
	RRA	4.10	0.06

Table 1.
Summary of ANOVA results for effects of prolonged sitting ($p<0.05$).

changes in the EMG signal during different working levels [23]. During low-level sustained muscle contractions, inconsistent evidence of fatigue development was observed between different muscle groups and across individuals [10]. Therefore, the analysis of EMG amplitude and median frequency as a measurement of muscle fatigue could lead to unreliable or conflicting results under low-level contractions. Existing evidence [11, 24], on the other hand, also illustrates the possibility of using traditional EMG methods to quantify muscle fatigue during low-level contractions as low as 2% MVC. However, these results were achieved from a relatively short duration with large inter-subject variations. Therefore, a sensitive method is needed to obtain reliable muscle fatigue measurements under these conditions of low-level sustained muscle contractions, i.e., prolonged sitting.

An alternative method to identify muscle fatigue is to combine muscle EMG with muscle stimulation technology. In this approach, an electrical stimulation pulse is sent to the target muscle to evoke an artificial muscle contraction, and the corresponding muscle stimulation response from these artificial contractions can be captured through surface EMG and other quantitative methods. In this method, muscle fatigue is defined as a significant change of observed muscle stimulation responses from the initial pre-fatigue status [25, 26]. Muscle fatigue has been identified using a single stimulation frequency [27, 28] or calculated as a decrement ratio of stimulation response results from high-frequency (50–100 Hz) and low-frequency (1–20 Hz) stimulation [26, 29]. While various stimulation frequencies have been used, low-frequency stimulation (LFS) usually creates stable stimulation responses and fatigue-induced changes [27]. Another benefit of using LFS is that it is less likely to cause muscle fatigue, and the level of discomfort is also low [28].

Therefore, in this chapter, a muscle stimulation method was further applied to determine the muscle fatigue results from prolonged sitting. All six participants completed a muscle stimulation trial after the initial MVC test and then repeated after the prolonged seated task, and the stimulation responses collected through both stimulation trials were compared to identify the potential muscle fatigue caused by the prolonged sitting.

Muscle stimulation responses were evoked using a dual-channel current-controlled muscle stimulator (Grass S88, AstroMed, RI) connected with a stimulus isolation unit (SIU5, AstroMed, RI) and a constant current unit (CCU1, AstroMed, RI). In this study, the MF muscle was selected to evaluate prolonged sitting induced muscle fatigue. The participant's skin around the MF muscle was appropriately prepared following the procedure described by [30]. After bilaterally placing the positive and negative stimulation electrodes (PALS, Axelgaard Manufacturing, CA) at the level of the rib cage bottom and the iliac crest, respectively, the most effective site for electrical stimulation was determined as suggested in [31] to determine appropriate stimulus intensity and electrode location for each participant. During the stimulation trial, participants were asked to sit in a customized fixture (**Figure 4**), with their upper body locked in a comfortable and relaxed upright sitting posture using a metal bar connected to their chest harness around the T8 level. A load cell (SM2000, Interface, AZ) was connected to the other end of the metal bar to collect the stimulation response (i.e., stimulation generated forces) generated by the artificial muscle contraction evoked by the stimulation. Muscle voluntary contractions were minimized by asking participants to relax their muscles and let the fixture hold their sitting postures. The muscle EMG were also monitored bilaterally to ensure minimal voluntary muscle contraction involved during the stimulation procedure. The stimulation train was repeated if the voluntary muscle contraction level monitored by surface EMG were greater than 5% of MVC. The fixture also has a height-adjustable seat pan to align the participant's trunk rotation center at the level of the L5/S1 joint in the sagittal plane. The participant's knee and ankle were also required to maintain a 90-degree using an adjustable footrest. While maintain such sitting posture, participants were also instructed to try to relax their muscles and eliminate potential movement during the data collection.

The overall experimental procedure was illustrated in **Figure 5**. Each participant completed one stimulation trial, starting with one conditioning train and three sampling trains, before and after the prolonged seat task. A conditioning

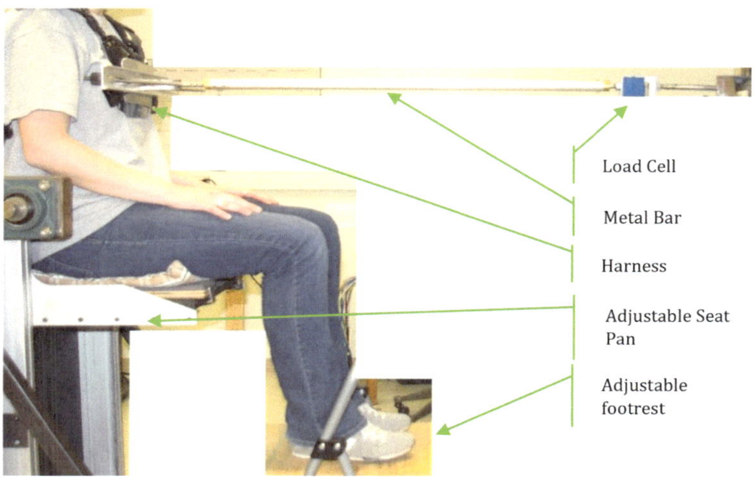

Figure 4.
Illustration of experimental fixture setup with a participant in an upright sitting posture.

train included stimulating muscles continuously at 2 Hz until a plateau and steady phases of measured muscle stimulation responses were observed. The duration of conditioning, i.e., the time-to-potentiation (t_p), is determined as the time at which the increasing rate of muscle stimulation response becomes zero. Immediately after the conditioning train, the same 2 Hz stimulation was applied again, and muscle stimulation responses were collected during three 9-second trains with a 10-second rest in between.

A repeated-measures analysis of variance (ANOVA) method was used to identify any significant changes in muscle stimulation response before and after the one hour of prolonged sitting.

Descriptive summaries of the stimulation response (i.e., stimulation generated forces) from two test trials are presented in **Figure 6**. Signs of muscle fatigue were clearly found in the measured stimulation response. Prolonged sitting resulted in a significant ($p = 0.03$) decrease in stimulation responses from the measured muscles.

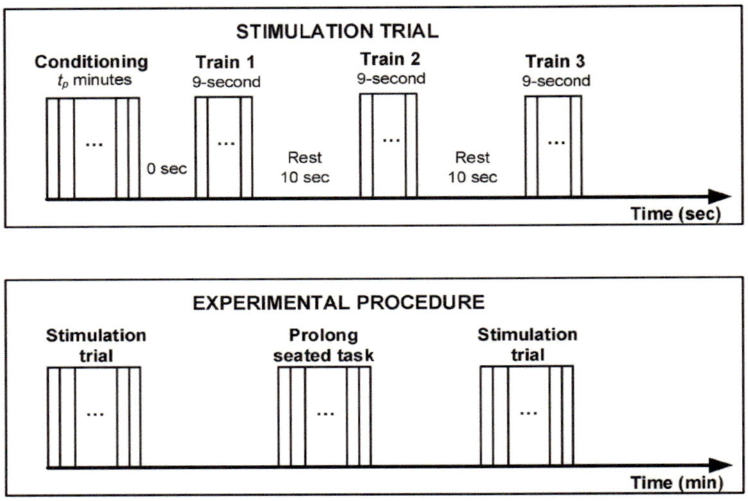

Figure 5.
Illustration of the overall experimental procedure. Conditioning: t_p minutes continuous stimulation at 2 Hz; train: 9-second stimulation at 2 Hz with a 10-second rest in between.

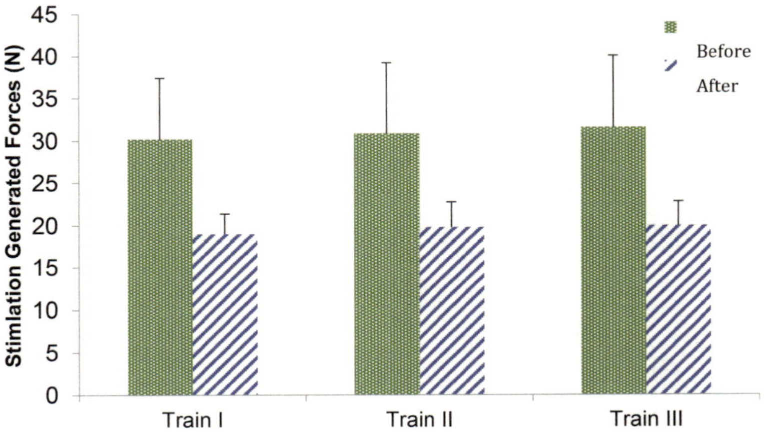

Figure 6.
Stimulation generated forces (mean and SD) collected among three trains before and after the prolonged seated task.

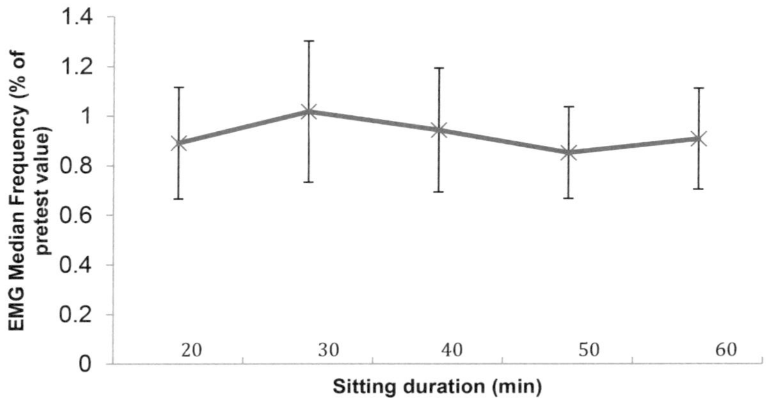

Figure 7.
Average EMG MPF of MF during the prolonged seated task.

As a comparison shown in **Figure 7**, the average EMG MPF of bilateral MF showed some signs of fatigue with a shifted MPF value, but the development of muscle fatigue was inconsistent over time, and the level of the observed shift was small.

3. Discussion and conclusions

Muscle fatigue was measured using EMG MPF, EMG amplitude, and muscle stimulation methods. In general, all three methods successfully captured the sign of muscle fatigue development through prolonged sitting. Consistency among these three measures supports that muscle fatigue indeed developed during the prolonged seated task.

EMG amplitude collected from 16 muscle groups showed a sign of increased amplitude toward the end of the sitting period. Two out of 16 muscles (i.e., LMF and LLTT) have significant increases in measured EMG amplitude, which in the absence of interference from external forces or movement may have been caused by muscle fatigue development over time. However, the EMG amplitude method did not detect any significant development of muscle fatigue over the rest of the 14 muscles, which may indicate the limited sensitivity of such methods in measuring muscle fatigue under prolonged sitting conditions. Furthermore, existing evidence also indicated that such EMG amplitude changes over a fatiguing task is also associated with the level of contraction, e.g., a task, which requires below 40% MVC, may show sign of EMG amplitude decrease [32], while other studies show increase of EMG amplitude during 40–50% MVC sustained contraction tasks [33, 34]. Therefore, using EMG amplitude alone may not be able to provide reliable estimation on muscle fatigue development.

EMG MPFs collected from four out of 16 muscles also showed signs of fatigue, but no general consistency was observed across all measured muscles. Some of the inconsistencies among various muscles in the measured MPFs may have been the result of the insensitivity of EMG in measuring low-load muscle fatigue. As shown in **Figure 2**, the average contraction level of most flexors and some extensors are between 2% and 5%. Since only a deficient level of muscle contractions are needed during the prolonged seated task, collected EMG signals may fall close to or even below the noise threshold, which may significantly affect the fatigue detection results derived from noisy EMG MPF. As a result, EMG amplitude and EMG MPF may only have limited capacity in measuring fatigue related muscle changes under such task conditions.

Another potential explanation could be linked to the functional differences between the trunk flexors and extensors. During the prolonged sitting, trunk extensors usually work as postural muscles that continuously contract to stabilize the sitting posture [5, 6]. Therefore, the observed decline of EMG MPF among three trunk extensors (ILL, LTT, and MF) was more substantial and could be used as a reasonable measurement of muscle fatigue caused by prolonged sitting. The decline of EMG MPF in the IO suggests that this muscle may also play an essential role in stabilizing the trunk posture during sitting, which is consistent with existing evidence [35]. All other muscles may have received only limited impacts from the prolonged seated task, or the actual fatigue could not be accurately measured using surface EMG during prolonged sitting.

Muscle fatigue measured by muscle stimulation, on the other hand, was more announced with a significant drop in measured stimulation responses across all three sampling trains. The same sign of fatigue was also observed in measured EMG amplitude and EMG MPF, but the magnitude of changes was small and inconsistent. Such results could indicate that muscle stimulation methods, compared to traditional EMG-based fatigue measurement methods, could provide more stable and visible results as a more sensitive method.

In summary, several EMG-based methods have been discussed in terms of their capabilities and limitations when used as ergonomic assessment methods to measure the effects of prolonged sitting. These outcomes were evident after one hour of continuous sitting. The effects of prolonged sitting have been successfully quantified by monitoring participants' muscle fatigue development. Current findings suggest that individuals who sit for prolonged periods can be at increased risk of cumulative disorder and injury, and various EMG-based methods can be used together to provide more reliable estimation and evaluation.

Conflict of interest

The author declares no sources of support or conflict of interest.

Author details

Bochen Jia
University of Michigan-Dearborn, Dearborn, Michigan, USA

*Address all correspondence to: bochenj@umich.edu

References

[1] Bureau of Labor Statistics, U.S. Department of Labor. Nonfatal Occupational Injuries and Illnesses Requiring Days Away from Work. 2018.

[2] Owen, N., Salmon, J., Koohsari, M. J., Turrell, G., & Giles-Corti, B. Sedentary behaviour and health: mapping environmental and social contexts to underpin chronic disease prevention. British Journal of Sports Medicine. 2014; 48(3), 174-177

[3] Chaffin, D. B., G. Andersson, et al. Occupational Biomechanics. New York, Wiley-Interscience Publication.1999.

[4] Pope, M. H., K. L. Goh, et al. Spine ergonomics. Annual Review of Biomedical Engineering. 2002; 4: 49-68.

[5] O'Sullivan, P. B., Mitchell, T., Bulich, P., Waller, R., & Holte, J. The relationship between posture and back muscle endurance in industrial workers with flexion-related low back pain. Manual Therapy, 2006; 11(4), 264-271.

[6] Nairn, B. C., Azar, N. R., & Drake, J. D. Transient pain developers show increased abdominal muscle activity during prolonged sitting. Journal of Electromyography and Kinesiology. 2013; 23(6):1421-7.

[7] Schinkel-Ivy, A., Nairn, B. C., & Drake, J. D. Investigation of trunk muscle co-contraction and its association with low back pain development during prolonged sitting. Journal of Electromyography and Kinesiology. 2013;23(4):778-86.

[8] Mork, P. J., & Westgaard, R. H., Back posture and low back muscle activity in female computer workers: a field study. Clinical Biomechanics. 2009; 24(2):169-75.

[9] Van Dieën, J. H., De Looze, M. P., & Hermans, V. Effects of dynamic office chairs on trunk kinematics, trunk extensor EMG and spinal shrinkage. Ergonomics. 2001; 44(7):739-50.

[10] Vøllestad, N. K. Measurement of human muscle fatigue. Journal of Neuroscience Methods. 1997; 74(2):219-27.

[11] Bernard, B. P., ed., Putz-Anderson, V., et al. Musculoskeletal Disorders and Workplace Factors: A Critical Review of Epidemiologic Evidence for Work-Related Musculoskeletal Disorders of the Neck, Upper Extremity, and Low Back. U.S. Department of Health and Human Services. 1997.

[12] Womersley, L., & May, S. Sitting posture of subjects with postural backache. Journal of Manipulative and Physiological tTherapeutics. 2006;29(3):213-8.

[13] McLean, L., & Goudy, N. Neuromuscular response to sustained low-level muscle activation: within- and between-synergist substitution in the triceps surae muscles. European Journal of Applied Physiology. 2004;91(2-3):204-16.

[14] van Dieën, J. H., Westebring-van der Putten, E. P., Kingma, I., & de Looze M. P. Low-level activity of the trunk extensor muscles causes electromyographic manifestations of fatigue in absence of decreased oxygenation. Journal of Electromyography and Kinesiology. 2009;19(3):398-406.

[15] McLean, L., Scott, R. N., et al. Measurement of muscle fatigue in the cervical and lumbar regions during prolonged sitting. Engineering in Medicine and Biology Society, 1997. Proceedings of the 19th Annual International Conference of the IEEE.

[16] Yoshizawa, N., Michida, N., Iname, C., & Furugori, S. Evaluation

of muscular fatigue after long-term sitting in automotive seat. JSAE Review. 2002;1(23):136-8.

[17] McGill, S. M. A myoelectrically based dynamic three-dimensional model to predict loads on lumbar spine tissues during lateral bending. Journal of Biomechanics. 1992;25(4):395-414.

[18] De Zee, M., Hansen, L., Wong, C., Rasmussen, J., & Simonsen, E. B. A generic detailed rigid-body lumbar spine model. Journal of Biomechanics. 2007;40(6):1219-27.

[19] Cholewicki, J., McGill, S. M., & Norman, R. W. Comparison of muscle forces and joint load from an optimization and EMG assisted lumbar spine model: towards development of a hybrid approach. Journal of Biomechanics. 1995; 28(3):321-31.

[20] Cholewicki J, van Dieën J, Lee AS, Reeves NP. A comparison of a maximum exertion method and a model-based, sub-maximum exertion method for normalizing trunk EMG. Journal of Electromyography and Kinesiology. 2011;21(5):767-73.

[21] Ng JK, Kippers V, Parnianpour M, Richardson CA. EMG activity normalization for trunk muscles in subjects with and without back pain. Medicine and Science in Sports and Exercise. 2002;34(7):1082.

[22] Potvin, J. R., Norman, R. W., & McGill, S. M. Mechanically corrected EMG for the continuous estimation of erector spinae muscle loading during repetitive lifting. European Journal of Applied Physiology and Occupational Physiology. 1996;74(1-2):119-32.

[23] Öberg. T., Sandsjö, L., Kadefors. R., & Larsson, S. E. Electromyographic changes in work-related myalgia of the trapezius muscle. European Journal of Applied Physiology and Occupational Physiology. 1992;65(3):251-7.

[24] Søgaard, K., Blangsted, A. K., Jørgensen, L. V., Madeleine, P., & Sjøgaard, G. Evidence of long term muscle fatigue following prolonged intermittent contractions based on mechano-and electromyograms. Journal of Electromyography and Kinesiology. 2003;13(5):441-50.

[25] Binder-Macleod S. A., & Snyder-Mackler, L. Muscle fatigue: clinical implications for fatigue assessment and neuromuscular electrical stimulation. Physical Therapy. 1993;73(12):902-10.

[26] Edwards, R. H., Hill, D. K., Jones D.A., & Merton, P. A. Fatigue of long duration in human skeletal muscle after exercise. The Journal of Physiology. 1977;272(3):769-78.

[27] Cooper, R. G., Edwards, R. H., Gibson, H., & Stokes, M. J. Human muscle fatigue: frequency dependence of excitation and force generation. The Journal of Physiology. 1988;397(1):585-99.

[28] Johnson, P. W., Lehman, S. L., & Rempel, D. M. Measuring low frequency fatigue with 2 Hertz stimulation. I. Stimulus-related potentiation effects. In Proceedings of 17th International Conference of the Engineering in Medicine and Biology Society 1995; (Vol. 2, pp. 1207-1208). IEEE.

[29] Jia B, Nussbaum MA, Agnew MJ. A Stimulation Method to Assess the Contractile Status of the Lumbar Extensors in a Seated Posture. Human Factors and Ergonomics in Manufacturing & Service Industries. 2015; 25(6):674-84.

[30] Cram J. R., & Rommen, D. Effects of skin preparation on data collected using an EMG muscle-scanning procedure. Biofeedback and Self-regulation. 1989;14(1):75-82.

[31] Karnes, J. L., Ed. Neuromuscular Electrical Stimulation: A Practical Guide. The Free Library. 2008.

[32] Seidel H, Beyer H, Bräuer D. Electromyographic evaluation of back muscle fatigue with repeated sustained contractions of different strengths. European journal of applied physiology and occupational physiology. 1987;56(5):592-602.

[33] Ng JK, Richardson CA, Jull GA. Electromyographic amplitude and frequency changes in the iliocostalis lumborum and multifidus muscles during a trunk holding test. Physical therapy. 1997;77(9):954-61.

[34] Holmström E, Moritz U, Andersson M. Trunk muscle strength and back muscle endurance in construction workers with and without low back disorders. Scandinavian journal of rehabilitation medicine. 1992;24(1):3-10.

[35] Snijders, C. J., Bakker, M. P., Vleeming, A., Stoeckart, R., & Stam, H. J. Oblique abdominal muscle activity in standing and in sitting on hard and soft seats. Clinical Biomechanics. 1995;10(2):73-8.

Chapter 4

Sedentary Behavior, Cardiovascular Risk and Importance of Physical Activity and Breaking-Up Sedentary Behavior

Imtiyaz Ali Mir

Abstract

Sedentary behavior (SB) is one of the common leading modifiable risk factor for cardiovascular (CV) morbidity and all-cause mortality. However, not much is known concerning the relationship between SB and CV risk factors. This chapter aimed to explore the scientific knowledge that examines the association between SB and CV risk factors and its association with the development of CVD. Besides, the focus on preventing the SB by avoiding prolonged sitting and breaking-up the extended periods of sitting, and participating in physical activity (PA) are usually highlighted in this chapter, explaining how these intervention protocols can reduce the burden of CVD due to SB. Regardless of the known benefits of both PA and taking frequent breaks when engaging in sedentary tasks, the adaptation of a physically active lifestyle has remained very low because of various reasons; habitual behavior, insufficient or lack of time, misconceptions of CVD related health benefits from PA. Thus, it is very important to break these barriers associated with PA and encourage the physically inactive population, especially those who practice prolonged sitting to actively participate in PA and break the prolonged sitting time with regular interval breaks. Therefore, promotion of PA and limiting the sedentary tasks which would lead to improved levels of cardiorespiratory fitness (CRF) and better quality of living is necessary among all age groups, gender and ethnicities to prevent many chronic illnesses, specifically CVD and its associated risks related to SB.

Keywords: sedentary behavior, cardiovascular disease risk, prolonged sedentary time, moderate-to-vigorous physical activity, cardiorespiratory fitness

1. Introduction

The advancement of sedentary behavior (SB) research in health science has increased rapidly which has led to numerous terminologies and definitions about SB. With this fast development, a standardized, clear, and common definition is to be formulated to address these issues. The "Sedentary Behaviour Study network" (SBSN) carried out a project to overcome this issue and developed a comprehensive conceptual model based on movement, structured around 24 hour period (**Figure 1**), and defines SB as "any waking behaviour in which the energy expenditure is low, generally ≤1.5 metabolic equivalents (MET's) while in sitting, reclining or lying position" [1]. The SBRN definition of SB includes two parts; posture and energy expenditure. The postural element is very easily operationalized and broadly utilized to determine SB by use of inclinometers, questionnaires, and direct observation, but dismisses the energetic part. Nevertheless, it requires to be mentioned that accelerometers usually measure movement rather than energy expenditure and represents an indirect approach to assess energy expenditure. Some of the common examples of SB include television (TV) viewing, sitting in the classroom, computer use, desk-based occupations, and passive commuting.

It is very important to emphasize that SB differs from physical inactivity (PI), in which an individual usually does not perform any of the recommended moderate-to-vigorous physical activity (MVPA). Although SB and PA are on the opposite ends of energy expenditure continuum, the inclusion of a postural element is a requirement for this to be considered sedentary, suggesting that this is a distinctive and unique behavior that can be intervened on. A person could be is actually physically active for the recommended 75–150 minutes of moderate PA each week or 150–300 minutes of vigorous PA every week [2], yet he or she may sit for several hours a day in a sedentary occupation or during their leisure time. The

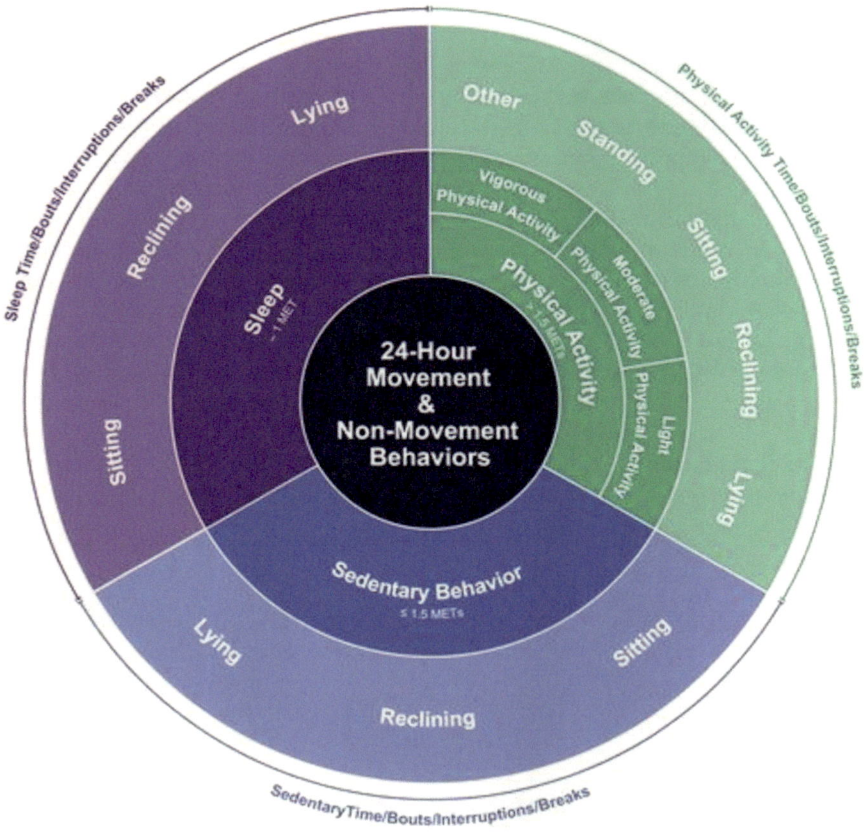

Figure 1.
"Movement-based terminology conceptual model based on 24 hours period. Picture organizes the movements that take place throughout the day, inner ring showing the energy expenditure and the outer ring displaying the posture. Courtesy - Tremblay et al. 2017.

adult population in the United States and the United Kingdom spend 60%–70% of the waking hours at sedentary activates, 25%–35% in light-intensity exercise, and the reminder little proportion of time on MVPA.

Time spent in SB is essential because it displaces the time spent in MVPA causing a decrease in overall PA energy expenditure. Displacement of 2 hours each day of light activity (2.5–3.0 MET's) by sedentary tasks (1.5 MET's) is predicted to decrease the PA energy expenditure by about 2 METs per hour each day or around the amount of energy expenditure while walking for 30 minutes per day. Research on PA and wellness has focused mostly on calculating the amount of time spent in PA carried out at 3 MET's or more, characterizing people that have no involvement in activates at such level as sedentary. Nevertheless, this explanation overlooks the considerable effect light-intensity PA can have daily on the overall expenditure energy [3] as well as the positive health-related outcome benefits by taking part in the light-intensity PA instead of simply sitting and doing nothing. Furthermore, although people could be both physically inactive and sedentary, additionally there is a higher chance of more time spent in sedentary tasks and PA to coexist. A good example could be an employee who jogs or bicycles to his or her workplace, but subsequently sits all day long at the workplace and spends many hours viewing TV at night after returning from work. Therefore, SB is not simply the absence of MVPA, but instead is a unique behavior with specific environment determinants and a variety of potentially distinctive wellness consequences.

Compared to previous generations, people are spending much more time in an environment which not merely restricts the PA, but also spent prolonged periods sitting at workplace, at home, in communities, and driving. Workplaces, schools, homes and common public areas are re-engineered in a manner that reduces body movements and muscle activity leading to dual influence on individuals behavior; move little and sit longer. Humans were made to locomote and take part in every form of manual labour on day to day basis. The recent change from a challenging and active life to one with only a few physical demands and challenges has been fast. The increased development of SB and its associated decrease in energy expenditure in the previous few years have become surprising. In the 1970s, 2 in 10 working people in America had been in occupations needing just light activity (primarily in sitting position), whereas 3 in 10 had been in occupations needing high energy expenditure like farming, manufacturing production, and construction [4]. By 2000, it was found more than 4 in 10 adults were in jobs that required light-to-moderate activity, whereas 2 in 10 had been at jobs that needed high energy expenditure. Furthermore, in the past 2 decades, the amount of screen time using computers and smartphones, playing video games and TV viewing has increased significantly. In 2003, about 6 in 10 working people used a computer at the job and 9 out of 10 children used a computer in schools and colleges. By 2016, more than 89% of households had a computer including a smartphone rendering it a common feature for everyday activity [5, 6].

Watching TV is associated with more than some other sedentary behaviors with higher CVD risk factors. It is hypothesized that watching TV results in lower energy expenditure than other sedentary activities like reading quietly in sitting, as a result of a slower resting metabolic rate. It is possible that watching TV requires less muscle contraction and activation than pursuits like driving, and this muscular inactivity is thought to be associated with a decrease in lipoprotein lipase [7], a protein that play an important role in managing lipid metabolism [8]. Therefore, more passive behavior of TV watching could have a strong association with higher CVD risk factors than various other sedentary activities because of reduced lipoprotein lipase. Another possible reason is that watching TV is connected with unhealthy nutritional habits, like decreased usage of fruits and vegetables and more intake of energy-dense food including fast food and sugar-sweetened beverages [9]. This may lead to increased snacking behavior while watching TV or expose people particularly young children to beverage and food advertising that attract them to make a harmful and unhealthy dietary choice [10]. Finally, a third feasible explanation is that people could be able to recall the period spent watching TV in comparison to the time allocated to other sedentary activities [11].

This chapter aimed to synthesize the scientific knowledge about the relationship between SB and CV risk factors and its association with the development of CVD. From the above findings it is very clear how people nowadays are spenting more time in SB, particularly extended period of time spent in watching TV, using computer and other electronic gadgets, administrative work, and passive commuting. All these sedentary tasks decrease the energy expenditure drastically and can negatively impact the health related outcome measures, and impose a higher risk of developing CVD and cardiometabolic disease. Furthermore, this chapter will explore the strategies that would help to prevent or minimize the SB by avoiding the prolonged sitting and breaking-up the extended periods of sitting, and engagement in physical activities, describing how these intervention protocols can reduce the burden of CVD due to SB.

2. Objective measurement of sedentary behavior

The uncertainty encircling the necessity for posture in the definition of SB poses challenges for measuring and evaluating measures of SB, as well as the difficulty in quantifying individual behavior. Most commonly used assessment options for SB consist of questionnaires, recalls, and behavioral logs, all of which possess methodological limitation of measurement errors. These assessment methods have fair to good reliability but reduced validity in comparison with criterion measures. However, objective assessment on SB can decrease measurement error and offer information regarding patterns of activities like time spent in sedentary tasks, breaks and MVPA. However, the drawbacks of objective based measurement include the cost of these objective tools, participant burden, converting data into the functional summary, devices failing to register position and intensity of some specific kind of activities (e.g. riding on a stationary bike), and insufficient information with regards to specific behavioral domains. Accelerometers (count the number of steps), heart-rate monitors, inclinometers along with other devices are used to offer an objective measurement of various variables such as intensity, volume, and frequency of a task that could be downloaded and converted into a purposeful activity interpretation. National Health and Nutrition Survey (NHANS) have been collecting accelerometer data from a large population of adults in the United States. The NHANS demonstrated that the degree of participation in MVPA's are lower and around 60% or even higher percentage of the adult population spent waking hours in sedentary activities [12, 13]. In a recently available validity study which was carried among 40 university employees aged 18–70 years, SB was evaluated by an accelerometer (<100 counts per minute [cpm]) that captured coded images by a very small wearable digital camera. The study demonstrated that some particular behaviors (watching TV, using computer and administrative routines) were properly classified utilizing the standard 100-cpm threshold by simpler accelerometry. Nevertheless, when tested for standing still position, it captured only 9% of the total time and generated <100-cpm 72% of that time, indicating that most of the time spent in standing will be categorized not as sedentary. However, scientists debate on what usually is the best-suited activity cut-off points to recognize time spent in sedentary tasks and time spent on the light-intensity activity. Besides, various cut-off points could be befitting populations of various ages, ethnic background, and adiposity status. **Figure 2** depicts a cluster heat map, displaying accelerometer information for a single individual during 1 week. The accelerometer value counts are recorded each minute, are usually represented by various colors. The darkish blue color represents accelerometer data information which is significantly less than the currently utilized, cut-off of 100-cpm for the sedentary tasks, and is mostly indicative of sitting behavior. Light blue through yellow color indicates some kind of light-to-moderate intensity activities, dark blue color indicates a very low level of expenditure of energy, and red color showing a high energy expenditure levels such as MVPA. What strikes the most is the degree to which this individual spends the time either in very light-intensity tasks as shown in pale-blue to white-color or mostly being sedentary as indicated by dark blue color.

Both self-reported and objective assessment methods could be essential to progress forward when quantifying the SB. Healy et al. [14] demonstrated that objective and self-reported sedentary behaviors are usually complementary and each provides distinct information. For instance, the TV viewing period was comparable for Mexican American citizens and non-Hispanic blacks (self-report), whereas overall time engaged in SB was shown to be increased in non-Hispanic blacks in comparison to Mexican Americans when assessed objectively. Therefore, understanding and possibly enhancing the reliability and validity of both self-report and objective assessment methods is a priory. Furthermore, due to the different information provided by each evaluation method, a better knowledge of the efficiency characteristics across both measurement approaches is needed.

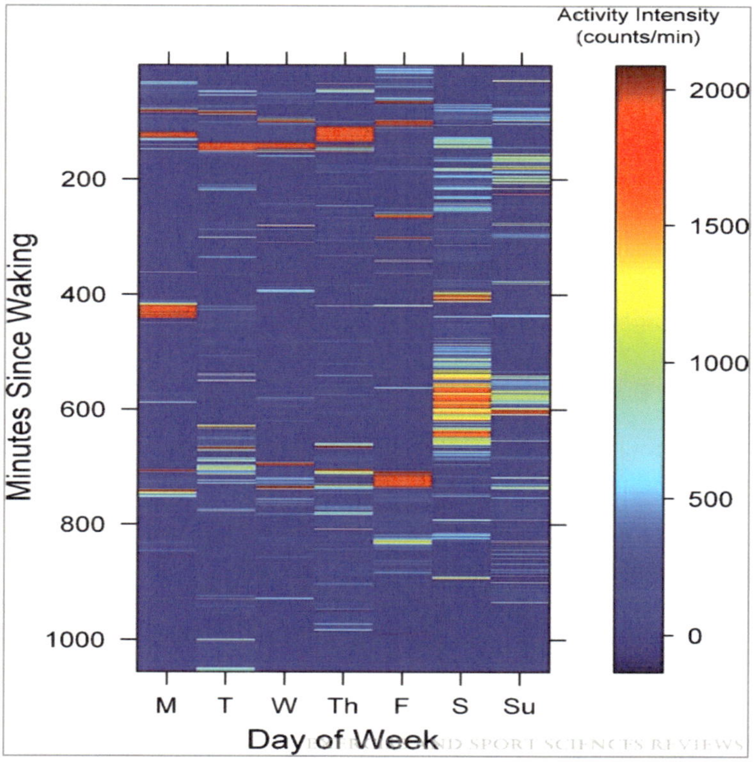

Figure 2.
1 week of accelerometer data - 31 minutes MVPA (> 1951 counts each minute), 71% waking hours being sedentary (> 100 counts every minute). Courtesy - Owen et al. 2010.

3. Sedentary behavior and risk of cardiovascular disease

Scientific research has been mostly centered on finding the association between SB and cardiometabolic morbidity and all-cause mortality. Little is known about the association between SB and higher cardiovascular (CV) risk and its advancement to CVD. The question that comes to mind is what are the possible mechanisms that contribute to the independent relation of SB with higher CVD morbidity and mortality? Probably the most likely and apparent explanation pertains to the influence of SB on risks associated with conventional CVD. Studies have established that in healthy adults, there is an association found between SB and higher conventional CV risk factors. Stamatakis et al. [15] reported the relationship of SB with conventional CV risks (Blood pressure [BP], high density lipoprotein cholesterol [HDL-C], WC, body mass index [BMI]) among 5948 healthy middle-age population. In another study, carried among 2328 young adult participants, prolonged sitting was observed to be independently and positively correlated with adiposity and heart rate and had a negative association with physical fitness as indicated by cardiorespiratory fitness (CRF) [16]. In a healthy population, very little scientific evidence is available on the relationship between SB and total cholesterol or low-density lipoprotein cholesterol (LDL-C) levels [17]. Nevertheless, evidence exists on the positive relationship between SB and triglycerides and HDL-C among the asymptomatic population which is mostly independent of PA [17, 18].

In addition to increased CV risks, SB is highly related to other adverse health-related outcomes, which include CV disease mortality, all-cause mortality, diabetes, increased insulin resistance, high BP, and obesity [15, 19, 20]. Researchers have noticed associations between SB and markers of CVD risk factors (high BP, decreased HDL-C, high triglyceride, and increased WC), which are usually independent of PA levels [15, 17]. Whitaker et al. [21] investigated the relationship between SB and higher CDV risks, authors discovered that the time spent in SB had deleterious associations with risks of CVD. The main factor of the association between SB and increased risk of CVD was time spent watching TV and other electronic gadgets. It was discovered that replacing time spent watching TV with any other kind of sedentary activities (use of the computer, sitting and reading, use of telephone, paperwork), led to a comparatively lower CDV risk. Besides, further findings revealed that the relationship of sedentary tasks with WC, glucose, insulin, and levels of triglyceride was consistent with results from the total CDV risk score, but a strong influence was found on triglyceride levels. Furthermore, the authors noticed that when computer time was replaced by using telephone or reading, this resulted in a high levels of BP. Another research study reported that watching TV had a positive association with numerous risks of CVD, such as BMI, waist to hip ratio, BP, total cholesterol, triglycerides and LDL-C [22]. This association was noticed in either gender and adjusted for age, alcohol consumption, cigarette smoking and dietary practices. There was no association found between PA and BP, LDL-C and total cholesterol. In fact, BP, LDL-C and total cholesterol had a strong association with PI, represented by TV viewing. A systematic review reported the risk of CVD disease in children and adolescents. A positive relationship was observed between screen-time (personal computer, video gaming, TV) and higher BP, reduced degrees of HDL-C, and higher degrees of LDL-C and triglycerides in children and adolescents. Even though not all of the studies support this association in the systematic review, there is growing evidence which indicates that SB is related with detrimental effects of health outcomes and there is a higher risk of developing CVD in children and adolescents. Additionally, not taking frequent breaks during the sedentary tasks and extended periods of sedentary bouts specifically watching TV and using other electronic gadgets actually compromise the cardiometabolic profile [23].

People with CV risk or disease seem to have an apparent relationship between SB and CV risk factors. In hypertensive patients, prolonged periods spent in SB were observed to be associated with higher BP readings [24]. Similarly, in the overweight and obese population, extended periods of sitting was found to have a positive and independent relationship with BP, a 14% increase in risk of developing hypertension with every additional one hour of sitting [25]. Beunza et al. [26] carried out a prospective cohort study among 6742 healthy university students over 40 months to assess the incidence of hypertension. Authors discovered that compared to non-sedentary adults, sedentary participants had a 48% increased risk of developing hypertension which was independent of PA.

A study among 945 participants in a cross-sectional examination found that after adjusting the BMI and BP, every 30 minutes of sedentary tasks were associated with a minimal ankle-brachial index [27]. In another research study among healthy participants, it was noticed that after adjusting for the vigorous PA, resting heart rate, metabolic syndrome, and adiposity, weekend breaks were positively connected with arterial stiffness [16]. These data sets provide proof that SB is positively associated with altered vascular functionality and structure. Further research is needed to explore and fully understand the connection between these complex relationships and examine if these detrimental effects on arterial health are independent of risk factors of CVD.

In short, it is evident from the growing scientific findings that there is a higher risk of CVD (high BP, arterial stiffness, increased BMI, higher levels of blood lipids, and deseased physical fitness) associated with SB as indictaed in **Figure 3**.

3.1 Effect of short periods of sitting on cardiovascular health

Recently studies have examined the effect on CV outcome measures related to short duration (3–6 hours) of continuous sitting. Padilla et al. [28] observed

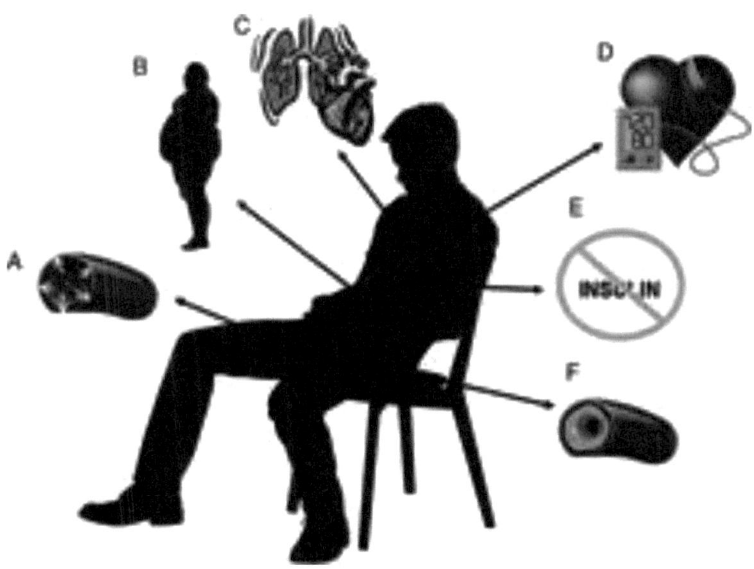

Figure 3.
Impact of sedentary behavior on risks associated with cardiovascular system: A. vasculature – Thickness and stiffness of intima-media increases. B. Anthropometric – Increased body mass index. C. Decrease in physical fitness (CRF). D. Increase in the blood pressure. E. Increase in insulin resistance. F. Increase in the blood lipids. Courtesy - Carter et al. 2017.

that continuous 3 hours of sitting resulted in an upsurge in the BP, together with a reduction in shear rate and blood flow in the popliteal artery. Similarly in another study, after 3 hours of continuous uninterrupted sitting, a reduction in the endothelial function of the superficial femoral artery (SFA) was observed, along with the simultaneous decrease in shear rate and antegrade [29]. These findings suggest that endothelial function in the lower limbs deteriorates with the practice of prolonged uninterrupted sitting. Compared to the lower limbs, uninterrupted sitting for 3 hours does not seem to have any effect on the endothelial function of upper limbs as no effect was reported in the brachial artery shear rate and endothelial function. Recently studies have explored the hypothesis that even little body movements, particularly the lower limb movements that are practiced during prolonged sitting prevent the impairment in the CV health outcomes. Larsen et al. [30] reported that during 7 hours of sitting, with a break given every 20 minutes to carry out light-to-moderate PA for 2 minutes, a significant reduction in both systolic and diastolic BP was seen. These findings point out that intervening on the SB may be appropriate and relevant, especially in a population with a high risk of CVD. Scientists have also examined the effect of regular breaks during prolonged sitting (5 hours to 3 days) on parameters such as lipids and triglycerides but did report any significant changes in any of these outcome measures [31, 32]. Perhaps longer duration break time coupled with some light-to-moderate PA is required to see the effect on these parameters. Because of the very limited information available on the impact of break time on uninterrupted prolonged sitting, further scientific research needs to be carried out to have a better understanding of the effects of break time and PA during prolonged sitting on CV risk factors.

The effect of break time and PA on uninterrupted prolonged sitting has also been investigated to find out its association with endothelial function. In normal healthy non-obese adults, after 3 hours of interrupted sitting, 5 minutes of light PA (walking on a treadmill at a speed of 2 miles per hour) every 60 minutes helped to prevent the reduction in the shear rate and dilation in SFA [29]. Another study also reported similar findings in a cohort of healthy young girls, in which the benefits of regular breaks and mild PA on SFA flow-mediated dilation were seen [33]. These findings suggest that sitting induced endothelial impairment can be offset when appropriate interventional strategies are implemented, particularly the use of low-intensity PA at regular intervals.

3.2 Effect of long periods of sitting on cardiovascular health

Currently, there is very little published literature available to support the claim that effects of long duration, acute exposure (usually more than 1 day) of SB on risk factors associated with higher CVD devlopment. Lyden et al. [34] evaluated effects on lipids and markers of insulin resistance in 10 healthy adults by imposing 7 days of prolonged sitting with little breaks in between. In comparison to the baseline, there was no change seen in fasting plasma lipids, BMI, and WC after 7 days of SB. But, when measured for 2 hours plasma insulin using oral glucose tolerance test and region under the curve were significantly increased after 7 days of prolonged sitting, indicating a detrimental capability of SB to lead to insulin resistance within 1 week [34]. In another study, the authors examined the effect of 3 days of intervention, using either 7 hours of sitting per day with 2 minutes light-intensity walks every 20 minutes or 7 hours per day of uninterrupted sitting without any breaks [31]. As measured by a mixed meal tolerance test, a significant decrease in glucose and insulin area under the curve was found after 3 days of uninterrupted sitting when compared with the group that was given breaks. As described above in this chapter, triglyceride levels did not differ between the 2 groups. Therefore, literature findings on short-term effects, usually between 3 to 7 days or immediate effects, between 3 to 6 hours of SB suggest the presence of quite significantly impaired insulin resistance, even in absence of such changes in the lipid levels. Research work carried out by Graves et al. [35] documented that using standing workstations in comparison to sitting workstations showed an average reduction of 90 minutes in sitting time every day over a period of 8 weeks. Further findings of a significant reduction in total cholesterol support the idea that extended periods of PI is required to cause an alteration in the lipid levels. To conclude, both short term and long term SB can alter vascular health such as endothelial function, peripheral blood flow, and BP.

Mechanisms underlying the SB induced vascular changes are thought to a result of haemodynamic stimuli, most probably the shear stress that causes structural and functional changes in vascular health [36]. Likewise, extended periods of uninterrupted sitting are found to be related to variations in the shear stress which could also induce vascular dysfunction. **Figure 4** summarizes the possible mechanisms associated with sitting induced risks of CVD. Hydrostatic pressure in the lower limbs is found to increase with prolonged sitting, specifically in the popliteal artery. When sitting for more than 3 hours without a break, a decrease in minimum, maximum and mean shear rate is observed in the popliteal artery [28]. Some studies have examined how alterations in shear can cause a decrease in the endothelial function related to extended periods of uninterrupted sitting. Investigations among young healthy adults revealed popliteal artery endothelial impairments caused by 3 hours of an extended period of sitting was effectively reduced by manipulating the popliteal artery perfusion via small fidgeting leg movements or by application of local heat [37, 38]. Both of these interventional strategies effectively prevented any decrease in mean shear which is associated with extended periods of uninterrupted sitting and appropriately prevented any decrease in endothelial function of the

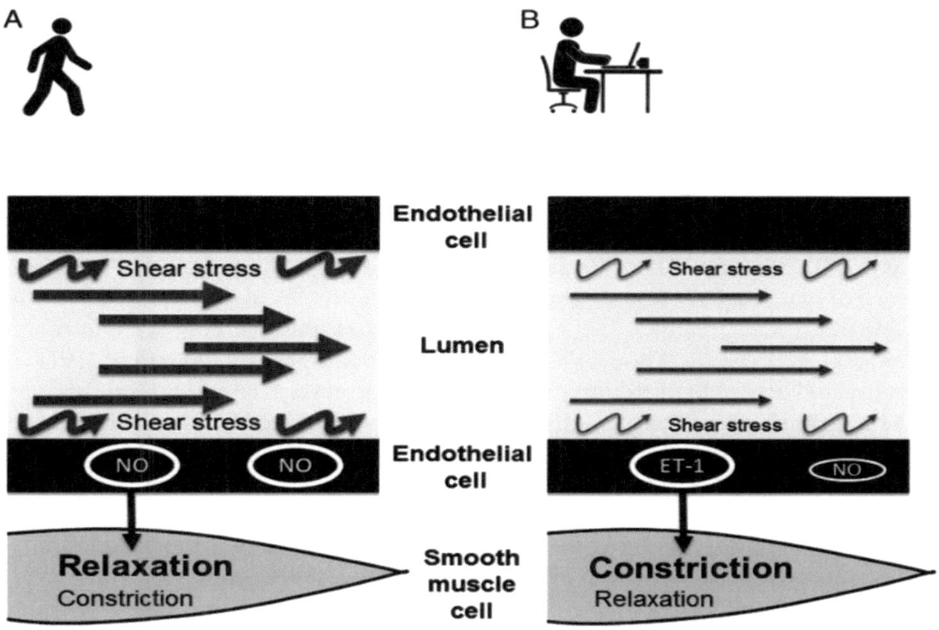

Figure 4.
Overview of mechanisms that mediate risk of cardiovascular disease in association with sedentary behavior: A. arterial structure and function while walking, increased shear stress and normal blood flow. B. Arterial structure and function after a period of SB, shear stress and blood flow is decreased, subsequently causing an increase in nitric oxide production leading to vascular dysfunction. Courtesy - Carter et al. 2017.

popliteal artery. It is believed that patterns of the shear may be equally important in addition of reduction in shear rate; it seems that shear patterns play an important role in maintaining the vascular function by increasing the endothelial function by activating the nitric oxide production or by preserving the antegrade shear stress; even though oscillatory and low shear stress can induce inflammation, increased oxidative stress and atherosclerosis [36].

The hypothesis related to changes in the shear rate and patterns is currently not well known. One of the possible reasons is that exposure to the prolonged periods of gravitational forces can elevate the hydrostatic pressure in the lower extremities, resulting in the pooling of venous blood followed by a reduction in the shear force and blood flow [39]. It has been observed that prolonged sitting causes an increase in calf circumference, reduced blood flow, and calf pooling [39]. Furthermore, an increase in the activity of the sympathetic nervous system and variations in the blood viscosity may also attribute to the alterations in the shear rate and patterns which can lead to further endothelial dysfunction [39]. All these factors may individually or in whole play a role in contributing to this relationship between prolonged sitting and dysfunction of vascular health.

4. Sedentary behavior and mortality

A nationwide cohort study in the United States revealed how sedentary time is strongly associated with all-cause mortality [40]. Over four years in a sample of 7985 middle-aged and elderly population, there had been 340 deaths reported overall. Further analysis demonstrated that longer SB with a sedentary time of more than 12 hours per day and sedentary bouts of more than 10 minutes per bout had the highest mortality risk [40]. However, the findings from a Canada fitness survey mortality follow up to underscore the adverse cardiometabolic health consequences associated with prolonged sitting. Those participants who spent most of the day sitting were seen to have a significantly poor long-term mortality outcome in comparison to those who reported spending less time sitting [41]. Further analysis showed these associations with mortality were consistent with overall sitting time measured across all levels of self-reported data of participants. Surprisingly, the relationship between sitting time and mortality was found to be stronger among those participants who were overweight and obese [41]. In another study during 6.5 years of follow-up, it was found that watching TV for a long time had a significant association with all-cause mortality rate and higher CVD mortality rate [42]. Every 1 hour increase of watching TV was seen to be associated with 11% higher risk of all-cause mortality and 18% greater risk of CVD mortality rates. Besides, compared to those who watched TV less (< 2 hours every day), there was a 80% higher risk of CVD mortality and a 46% high risk of all-cause mortality among those who watched TV 4 hours or more every day. Both these risks were found to be independent of conventional risk factors like BP, cholesterol, smoking, WC, and diet indicating a strong relationship between SB and its detrimental effects on CV and overall health. In another study in the United States, the authors examined the relationship of SB with CVD mortality outcomes based on 21 years of follow up among 7744 participants aged 20–89 years. A total of 377 deaths were reported in this study. It was observed that TV time and time spent in commuting and combined time spent in these 2 sedentary activates had a strong positive association with increased CVD deaths even after age-adjustment. Compared with those who reported spending less than 4 hours every week sitting in automobiles, an 82% greater risk of CVD mortality was seen in those who reported spending more than 10 hours every week in passive commuting. Similarly, those who spent more than 23 hours per week of combined automobile time and TV time had a 64% higher risk of dying from CVD compared to those who spent less than 11 hours every week [20].

To combat all these adverse health-related outcome risks associated with SB, recently a major focus has been directed at making health promotion a priority, including the promotion to reduce the sitting time and to take frequent breaks, in addition to participate in PA to improve the levels of CRF.

5. Breaking-up long periods of sedentary behavior and engaging in physical activity

It is believed that most often serious efforts are required from the people to make even smaller changes in the health behavior to become a part of their lifestyle. With regards to this, interventional protocols that promote healthy behaviors should be easy to follow, simple, recognizable, and not require much energy from a cognitive perspective. Because prolonged sitting is regarded to be highly habitual, the interventional approaches used should be able to instantly elicit a response of breaking and getting up and thus decreasing the prolonged sitting time. Since prolonged sitting is considered to extremely habitual, with little if any conscious planning and processing compared to PA, which requires higher degrees of planning and mental processing. Thus it is easy to express that SB is different from PA based on the above explanation.

Scientific data has provided evidence that SB is highly associated with health risks (e.g. high BP, increased levels of triglycerides, lower DHL-C, arterial stiffness, and increased BMI and WC) regardless of the PA levels [15–17]. This shows that prolonged periods of sitting cannot be compensated by just 30 minutes of MVPA and a shift in the scientific focus has been suggested to include the physiology of sedentary inactivity together with exercise when considering to address the health issues related to SB [8, 31]. If a day is divided into periods of SB, light PA, and MVPA, it can be seen that very little time is spent on light PA and MVPA and a large period is spent on sedentary activates like TV viewing, use of computer and other electronic gadgets and passive commuting. Besides, if a person tries to reduce the SB, that time is mostly spent on doing light PA rather than MVPA. Thus, it makes a lot of sense to focus and target the SB as important health behavior.

Interventional approaches should promote a healthy lifestyle in addition of including the MVPA and simultaneously a major focus should be on reducing and breaking the prolonged sedentary time [43]. The reason for limiting the sitting time is that all sedentary activities evoke a catabolic response which suppresses the skeletal muscle lipoprotein activity [7]. Even though little evidence is available with regards to the thresholds for the prolonged sitting time or when exactly sitting should be interrupted before it can evoke the detrimental health consequences, it is suggested that when short breaks are taken frequently during prolonged sitting, it can help to prevent these detrimental health outcomes [29, 30, 32]. Recently in a systematic review, authors examined the experimental and epidemiological studies and concluded that breaking up prolonged sitting can generate positive effects on metabolic-related health outcomes, even though the type, intensity and frequency of PA were different for participants based on their characteristics, particularly with regards to their habitual PA levels in each study included in the review [44]. By looking at the healthy physiological responses that the body can generate by simply standing up and breaking the prolonged sitting, people with morbidity which are related to lifestyle (SB), may be able to benefit more by taking regular breaks and decreasing the prolonged sitting time [45].

5.1 American College of Sports Medicine guidelines on reducing sedentary behavior

In our current contemporary time, we cannot completely eliminate the time spent in sedentary behaviors, but breaking-up the prolonged sitting using simple activities such as standing or walking can be very helpful at preventing the deleterious health-related outcomes, especially minimizing the higher CVD risk associated with SB. In line with this, the American College of Sports Medicine recommends to adopt an active action plan both at workplace and home to break-up or reduce prolonged periods of sitting, which is summarized in **Table 1** [46].

5.2 World Health Organization (WHO 2020) guidelines on sedentary behavior and physical activity

World Health Organization (WHO 2020) has revised the guidelines on PA and SB for all age groups including people that live with chronic morbidity or disability. It is stated that for all age groups doing some PA is always better than doing no PA at all [2]. If people are physically inactive and living a sedentary life, they should begin with PA that is small in amount and of light intensity, then slowly increasing the intensity, frequency, and time duration over time. The following

Active action plan ideas for work	Active action plan ideas for daily life
1. Take a walk break every time you take a coffee or tea break. 2. Do some leisurely walking with colleagues after you eat lunch together. 3. Stand up and move whenever you have a drink of water. 4. Whenever possible stand up as opposed to sitting down. 5. Stand up and talk on phone conversations. 6. Stop at the park on your way home from work and take a walk. 7. Walk to a co-workers desk instead of emailing or calling him/her 8. Walk briskly when headed To meetings. 9. Take the stairs whenever you can. 10. Take the long route to the restroom. 11. Schedule walking meetings with colleagues. 12. Schedule short breaks into your electronic calendar as reminders to above. 13. Every 45 minutes to one hour, do some squats, lunges, upper body stretches, shoulder rolls.	1. Take a family walk after dinner. 2. Get a pedometer and start tracking your steps. Progress to 10,000 steps or more a day. 3. Walk your dog daily. 4. Replace those Sunday drives with Sunday walks. 5. Wen watching TV, stand up and move with every commercial break. 6. Walk up and down escalators instead of just riding them 7. Walk fast when doing errands. 8. Pace the sidelines at your kids' athletic games. 9. Walk up and down the shopping aisles at the store before you shop. 10. Pick up a new active hobby, such as cycling or hiking. 11. After reading six pages of a book, get up and move a little. 12. Try standing and moving whenever you are talking on a cell phone. 13. Play with your kids 15–30 minutes a day. 14. Dance to your favorite inspiring music selections. 15. Walk briskly in the mall.c

Sit less and move more: Len Kravitz, and Chantal a. Vella (ACSM).

Table 1.
American College of Sports Medicine Information on reducing sedentary behavior.

sub-heading will cover the recommendations on PA and SB for children and adolescents, adults, and elderly including those who live with chronic conditions/ disabilities in detail.

5.2.1 WHO 2020 recommendations for children and adolescents aged 5–17 years

In this population, PA confers benefits when it comes to physical fitness (CRF and muscle strength), cardiometabolic wellness (BP, dyslipidemia, glucose and insulin tolerance), bone health, cognitive functions like academic performance, and executive function, and decreased adiposity. It is suggested that this population should take part in moderate PA of at least 60 minutes every day across the week, with exercises mainly aerobic. Vigorous PA and exercises that target muscles and bones to increase the strength of these tissues should also be included at least 3 days every week. The research evidence suggests that there is a strong association between adverse health-related outcomes and SB, particularly between watching TV or recreational screen time with adverse health consequences in children and adolscents [2]. Therefore, very limited sedentary time should be allowed for this age group.

5.2.2 WHO 2020 recommendations for adults aged 18–64 years including people that have chronic conditions and disability

In grown-ups, PA confers advantages to all-cause mortality, CVD mortality, incident hypertension, incident type 2 diabetes and measures of adiposity. Recommendations for adults include 150–300 minutes of moderate-intensity PA, aerobic in nature 75–150 minutes of vigorous PA or combination of equivalent volumes of MVPA throughout the week. In addition, adults must also do muscle strengthening exercises at MVPA involving major muscle groups at least 2 or more days every week. Furthermore, evidence on effect of SB on health outcomes provide a strong support that prolonged sedentary time should be limited by adults [2].

5.2.3 WHO 2020 recommendations for older adults aged 65 years and above including people that have chronic conditions and disability

In this population, PA is beneficial in preventing falls and falls-related injuries and declines in bone health and functional ability. It is suggested that older people should follow the same guidelines as recommended for adults. In addition, the elderly should also engage in varied multicomponent PA that emphasizing strengthening exercises and functional training at the moderate-to-high intensity on 3 or even more days weekly. The recommendations on SB apply to this group in the same way as adults [2].

5.3 Australian guidelines on sedentary behavior and physical activity

Australian guidelines on SB and PA are supported by strong evidence and considers the relationship between PA (e.g. type of PA, intensity, frequency, and duration) and outcome indicators of health, including the risk of chronic diseases and obesity.

The association between SB and outcome indicators of health, including the risk of chronic disease and obesity [47]. Like WHO 2020 guidelines, Australian guidelines on PA and SB are divided based on different age groups.

5.3.1 Recommendations from birth to 5 years

Most of the waking hours of this group should be playful, engaging them in a variety of activities.

Infants from birth to 1 year: PA encouraged for this age group should be done under supervision, mostly floor-based activities of play conducted in safe environment. For infants that are not yet mobile, 30 minutes of tummy time period, which includes reaching, grasping, puling, pressing and crawling during awaking hours throughout the day [47].

Toddlers aged one to 1-2 years: For this group, it is recommended to carry out 180 minutes of varieties of PA, which include 60 minutes of energetic play like jumping, kicking, throwing and running during awaking hours throughout the day [47].

Small children aged 3-5 years: They should not be restrained in strollers or car seats for more than one hour or allowed to sit for prolonged time. Screen time spent in sedentary tasks (watching TV, playing with electronic gadgets) should not be more than one hour based on twenty four hour time period. When these children are sedentary, parents or caregivers should build a playful relationships with them through routines like singing, reading, storytelling using puzzles etc. [47].

5.3.2 Recommendations of young children and young people aged 5–17 years

This particular population ought to achieve the suggested and recommended low levels of SB and high levels of PA for optimal health benefits [47].

Guidelines on Physical Activity:

- 60 minutes or higher aerobic MVPA each day.
- Variety of several hours of light PA.
- Vigorous PA and strengthening workouts that target major muscle groups and bones ought to be included at least 3 times per week.
- Replacing sedentary time with additional MVPA to accomplish greater benefits of health [47].

Guidelines on Sedentary Behavior:

- Whenever possible breaking up prolonged periods of sedentary behavior.
- Not more than 2 hours to be spent on sedentary screen time.
- Emphasis on encouraging the positive social interactions when using electronic devices that are used for screen time [47].

5.3.3 Recommendations for adults aged 18–64 years

Guidelines on Physical Activity:

- All adults should take part in some type of PA, regardless of their age.
- Those who are beginning to engage in a new PA or those who were previously active but have stopped, shall start at a rate that is easily manageable and slowly build-up to the recommended levels.
- Adults should be active in many ways, participating in a wide range of PA that includes fitness, strength, flexibility and balance.

- They are encouraged to accumulate at least 30 minutes of moderate intensity PA, preferably every day.
- Older adults who had been enjoying vigorous PA of lifetime, shall continue to do so in a manner that is suited for their capacity, provided they abide by the recommended safety procedures and recommendations [47].

Guidelines on Sedentary Behavior:

- Whenever possible breaking-up prolonged sitting.
- Reduce the time spent in prolonged sitting [47].

5.3.4 Recommendations for older adults aged 64 years and above

For this population, being physically active for 30 minutes is achievable. In addition, their health and wellbeing can be improved further if a little increase in the recommended PA is achieved [47].

Guidelines on Physical Activity:

- If currently inactive, start with some light exercises and gradually target the recommended quantity.
- Encouraged to be physically active on most of the day, every week.
- 150–300 minutes of MVPA or 75–150 minutes of vigorous PA, or combined equivalent of MVPA, every week.
- Strengthening exercises, at least 2 times per week targeting major muscles groups of the body [47].

Guidelines on Sedentary Behavior:

The guidelines for SB are the same as recommended for adults, which includes minimizing the prolonged sitting time and taking frequent breaks whenever possible during sedentary tasks [47].

6. Conclusion

SB is a habitual behavior that can be managed effectively when appropriate interventional strategies are employed. If not ponder upon, it can lead to detrimental health consequences. Evidence strongly supports and recommends minimizing the sedentary time and taking regular breaks in between the sedentary tasks, in addition of incorporating the MVPA to decrease the CVD risks and compromising metabolic health. The higher risk of CVD mortality and morbidity and all-cause mortality is independent of PA levels in individuals who engage in longer periods of SB. Therefore, in addition to participating in recommended PA guidelines, equally important is to break-up prolonged sitting and reduce the time spent in sedentary tasks like watching TV, using the computer and other electronic gadgets, and passive commuting, which would lead to improved levels of CRF and better quality of life in all age groups, gender, race, and ethnicities.

Acknowledgements

I would to thank Universiti Tunku Abdul Rahamn for giving me enough time to complete this book chapter, without which it would have not been possible to complete this task.

Conflict of interest

"The author declare no conflict of interest."

Notes/thanks/other declarations

I would also like to thank my beloved wife, Shanilla Shaheen for supporting and encouraging me to write and complete this book chapter.

Author details

Imtiyaz Ali Mir
Faculty of Medicine and Health Sciences, Universiti Tunku Abdul Rahman, Bandar, Sunagi Long, Kajang, Selangor, Malaysia

*Address all correspondence to: imtiyaz2204@yahoo.com

References

[1] Tremblay MS, Aubert S, Barnes JD, Saunders TJ, Carson V, Latimer-Cheung AE, et al. Sedentary Behavior Research Network (SBRN) – Terminology Consensus Project process and outcome. Int J Behav Nutr Phys Act [Internet]. 2017 Jun 10 [cited 2020 Dec 15];14. Available from: https://www.ncbi.nlm.nih.gov/pmc/articles/PMC5466781/

[2] Bull FC, Al-Ansari SS, Biddle S, Borodulin K, Buman MP, Cardon G, et al. World Health Organization 2020 guidelines on physical activity and sedentary behaviour. Br J Sports Med. 2020 Dec 1;54(24):1451-62.

[3] Donahoo WT, Levine JA, Melanson EL. Variability in energy expenditure and its components. Curr Opin Clin Nutr Metab Care. 2004 Nov;7(6):599-605.

[4] Brownson RC, Boehmer TK, Luke DA. Declining rates of physical activity in the United States: what are the contributors? Annu Rev Public Health. 2005;26:421-43.

[5] US Census Bureau. Computer and Internet Use in the United States: October 2009 [Internet]. The United States Census Bureau. [cited 2020 Dec 15]. Available from: https://www.census.gov/data/tables/2009/demo/computer-internet/computer-use-2009.html

[6] US Census Bureau. Computer and Internet Use in the United States: 2016 [Internet]. The United States Census Bureau. [cited 2020 Dec 15]. Available from: https://www.census.gov/library/publications/2018/acs/acs-39.html

[7] Bey L, Hamilton MT. Suppression of skeletal muscle lipoprotein lipase activity during physical inactivity: a molecular reason to maintain daily low-intensity activity. J Physiol. 2003 Sep 1;551(Pt 2):673-82.

[8] Hamilton MT, Hamilton DG, Zderic TW. Role of Low Energy Expenditure and Sitting in Obesity, Metabolic Syndrome, Type 2 Diabetes, and Cardiovascular Disease. Diabetes. 2007 Nov 1;56(11):2655-67.

[9] Hobbs M, Pearson N, Foster PJ, Biddle SJH. Sedentary behaviour and diet across the lifespan: an updated systematic review. Br J Sports Med. 2015 Sep;49(18):1179-88.

[10] Harris JL, Bargh JA, Brownell KD. Priming effects of television food advertising on eating behavior. Health Psychol Off J Div Health Psychol Am Psychol Assoc. 2009 Jul;28(4):404-13.

[11] Clark BK, Sugiyama T, Healy GN, Salmon J, Dunstan DW, Owen N. Validity and reliability of measures of television viewing time and other non-occupational sedentary behaviour of adults: a review. Obes Rev Off J Int Assoc Study Obes. 2009 Jan;10(1):7-16.

[12] Nielsen Company Three Screen Report. Q1 2010 Report . What Consumers Watch [Internet]. [cited 2020 Dec 15]. Available from: https://www.nielsen.com/us/en/insights/article/2010/what-consumers-watch-nielsens-q1-2010-three-screen-report/

[13] Matthews CE, Chen KY, Freedson PS, Buchowski MS, Beech BM, Pate RR, et al. Amount of time spent in sedentary behaviors in the United States, 2003-2004. Am J Epidemiol. 2008 Apr 1;167(7):875-81.

[14] Healy GN, Wijndaele K, Dunstan DW, Shaw JE, Salmon J, Zimmet PZ, et al. Objectively measured sedentary time, physical activity, and metabolic risk: the Australian Diabetes, Obesity and Lifestyle Study (AusDiab). Diabetes Care. 2008 Feb;31(2):369-71.

[15] Stamatakis E, Hamer M, Tilling K, Lawlor DA. Sedentary time in relation

to cardio-metabolic risk factors: differential associations for self-report vs accelerometry in working age adults. Int J Epidemiol. 2012 Oct;41(5):1328-37.

[16] Huynh QL, Blizzard CL, Sharman JE, Magnussen CG, Dwyer T, Venn AJ. The cross-sectional association of sitting time with carotid artery stiffness in young adults. BMJ Open. 2014 Mar 6;4(3):e004384.

[17] Brocklebank LA, Falconer CL, Page AS, Perry R, Cooper AR. Accelerometer-measured sedentary time and cardiometabolic biomarkers: A systematic review. Prev Med. 2015 Jul;76:92-102.

[18] Shuval K, Finley CE, Barlow CE, Gabriel KP, Leonard D, Kohl HW. Sedentary behavior, cardiorespiratory fitness, physical activity, and cardiometabolic risk in men: the cooper center longitudinal study. Mayo Clin Proc. 2014 Aug;89(8):1052-62.

[19] Thorp AA, Owen N, Neuhaus M, Dunstan DW. Sedentary Behaviors and Subsequent Health Outcomes in Adults: A Systematic Review of Longitudinal Studies, 1996-2011. Am J Prev Med. 2011 Aug 1;41(2):207-15.

[20] Warren TY, Barry V, Hooker SP, Sui X, Church TS, Blair SN. Sedentary behaviors increase risk of cardiovascular disease mortality in men. Med Sci Sports Exerc. 2010 May;42(5):879-85.

[21] Whitaker KM, Buman MP, Odegaard AO, Carpenter KC, Jacobs DR, Sidney S, et al. Sedentary Behaviors and Cardiometabolic Risk: An Isotemporal Substitution Analysis. Am J Epidemiol. 2018 Feb;187(2):181-9.

[22] Aadahl M, Kjær M, Jørgensen T. Influence of time spent on TV viewing and vigorous intensity physical activity on cardiovascular biomarkers. The Inter 99 study. Eur J Cardiovasc Prev Rehabil. 2007 Oct 1;14(5):660-5.

[23] Canabrava KLR, Amorim PR dos S, Miranda VPN, Priore SE, Franceschini S do CC, Canabrava KLR, et al. SEDENTARY BEHAVIOR AND CARDIOVASCULAR RISK IN CHILDREN: A SYSTEMATIC REVIEW. Rev Bras Med Esporte. 2019 Oct;25(5):433-41.

[24] Gerage AM, Benedetti TRB, Farah BQ, Santana F da S, Ohara D, Andersen LB, et al. Sedentary Behavior and Light Physical Activity Are Associated with Brachial and Central Blood Pressure in Hypertensive Patients. PLoS ONE [Internet]. 2015 Dec 30 [cited 2020 Dec 18];10(12). Available from: https://www.ncbi.nlm.nih.gov/pmc/articles/PMC4696789/

[25] King WC, Chen J-Y, Courcoulas AP, Mitchell JE, Wolfe BM, Patterson EJ, et al. Objectively-measured sedentary time and cardiometabolic health in adults with severe obesity. Prev Med. 2016 Mar 1;84:12-8.

[26] Beunza JJ, Martínez-González MA, Ebrahim S, Bes-Rastrollo M, Núñez J, Martínez JA, et al. Sedentary behaviors and the risk of incident hypertension: the SUN Cohort. Am J Hypertens. 2007 Nov;20(11):1156-62.

[27] Parsons TJ, Sartini C, Ellins EA, Halcox JPJ, Smith KE, Ash S, et al. Objectively measured physical activity and sedentary behaviour and ankle brachial index: Cross-sectional and longitudinal associations in older men. Atherosclerosis. 2016 Apr;247:28-34.

[28] Padilla J, Sheldon RD, Sitar DM, Newcomer SC. Impact of acute exposure to increased hydrostatic pressure and reduced shear rate on conduit artery endothelial function: a limb-specific response. Am J Physiol Heart Circ Physiol. 2009 Sep;297(3):H1103-1108.

[29] Thosar SS, Bielko SL, Mather KJ, Johnston JD, Wallace JP. Effect of prolonged sitting and breaks in sitting

time on endothelial function. Med Sci Sports Exerc. 2015 Apr;47(4):843-9.

[30] Larsen RN, Kingwell BA, Sethi P, Cerin E, Owen N, Dunstan DW. Breaking up prolonged sitting reduces resting blood pressure in overweight/obese adults. Nutr Metab Cardiovasc Dis NMCD. 2014 Sep;24(9):976-82.

[31] Larsen RN, Kingwell BA, Robinson C, Hammond L, Cerin E, Shaw JE, et al. Breaking up of prolonged sitting over three days sustains, but does not enhance, lowering of postprandial plasma glucose and insulin in overweight and obese adults. Clin Sci Lond Engl 1979. 2015 Jul;129(2):117-27.

[32] Peddie MC, Bone JL, Rehrer NJ, Skeaff CM, Gray AR, Perry TL. Breaking prolonged sitting reduces postprandial glycemia in healthy, normal-weight adults: a randomized crossover trial. Am J Clin Nutr. 2013 Aug;98(2):358-66.

[33] McManus AM, Ainslie PN, Green DJ, Simair RG, Smith K, Lewis N. Impact of prolonged sitting on vascular function in young girls. Exp Physiol. 2015 Nov;100(11):1379-87.

[34] Lyden K, Keadle SK, Staudenmayer J, Braun B, Freedson PS. Discrete features of sedentary behavior impact cardiometabolic risk factors. Med Sci Sports Exerc. 2015 May;47(5):1079-86.

[35] E. F. Graves L, C. Murphy R, Shepherd SO, Cabot J, Hopkins ND. Evaluation of sit-stand workstations in an office setting: a randomised controlled trial. BMC Public Health. 2015 Nov 19;15(1):1145.

[36] Johnson BD, Mather KJ, Wallace JP. Mechanotransduction of shear in the endothelium: basic studies and clinical implications. Vasc Med Lond Engl. 2011 Oct;16(5):365-77.

[37] Restaino RM, Walsh LK, Morishima T, Vranish JR, Martinez-Lemus LA, Fadel PJ, et al. Endothelial dysfunction following prolonged sitting is mediated by a reduction in shear stress. Am J Physiol Heart Circ Physiol. 2016 Mar 1;310(5):H648-653.

[38] Morris JN, Crawford MD. Coronary Heart Disease and Physical Activity of Work. Br Med J. 1958 Dec 20;2(5111):1485-96.

[39] Restaino RM, Holwerda SW, Credeur DP, Fadel PJ, Padilla J. Impact of prolonged sitting on lower and upper limb micro- and macrovascular dilator function. Exp Physiol. 2015 Jul 1;100(7):829-38.

[40] Diaz KM, Howard VJ, Hutto B, Colabianchi N, Vena JE, Safford MM, et al. Patterns of sedentary behavior and mortality in U.S. middle-aged and older adults: A national cohort study. Ann Intern Med. 2017 Oct 3;167(7):465-75.

[41] Katzmarzyk PT, Church TS, Craig CL, Bouchard C. Sitting time and mortality from all causes, cardiovascular disease, and cancer. Med Sci Sports Exerc. 2009 May;41(5):998-1005.

[42] Dunstan DW, Barr ELM, Healy GN, Salmon J, Shaw JE, Balkau B, et al. Television viewing time and mortality: the Australian Diabetes, Obesity and Lifestyle Study (AusDiab). Circulation. 2010 Jan 26;121(3):384-91.

[43] Yates T, Wilmot EG, Khunti K, Biddle S, Gorely T, Davies MJ. Stand up for your health: Is it time to rethink the physical activity paradigm? Diabetes Res Clin Pract. 2011 Aug 1;93(2):292-4.

[44] Benatti FB, Ried-Larsen M. The Effects of Breaking up Prolonged Sitting Time: A Review of Experimental Studies. Med Sci Sports Exerc. 2015 Oct;47(10):2053-61.

[45] Lee I-M, Shiroma EJ, Lobelo F, Puska P, Blair SN, Katzmarzyk PT. Effect of physical inactivity on major non-communicable diseases worldwide: an analysis of burden of disease and life expectancy. The Lancet. 2012 Jul 21;380(9838):219-29.

[46] ACSM's Guidelines for Exercise Testing and Prescription. Physical Activity Guidelines Resources [Internet]. [cited 2020 Dec 15]. Available from: https://www.acsm.org/read-research/trending-topics-resource-pages/physical-activity-guidelines

[47] Australian Government: Department of Health. Australia's Physical Activity and Sedentary Behaviour Guidelines and the Australian 24-Hour Movement Guidelines [Internet]. Australian Government Department of Health; 2019 [cited 2020 Dec 21]. Available from: https://www1.health.gov.au/internet/main/publishing.nsf/Content/health-pubhlth-strateg-phys-act-guidelines

Chapter 5

How to Reduce Sedentary Behavior at All Life Domains

Olga López Torres, Pablo Lobo, Valeria Baigún and Gabriela F. De Roia

Abstract

Lifestyle has changed in the last century increasingly promoting sedentary behaviors. Prolonged sitting time is related to increased all-cause mortality risk. Therefore, scientific research aimed at understanding the effects of sitting on health has increased to find effective interventions that can be carried out in life domains (study, work, transport, and free time). The interaction between physical activity and sitting time plays a key role in the development of strategies to promote physical activity practice and reduce sedentary behavior. Accepting that the modern societies incite to spend long periods seated, the aim seems to find a balance between all the areas during the 24 h of the day. Maintaining sleep time, reducing screen leisure time to 3 h/day, and breaking prolonged sedentary time for 2–3 min every 30 min-1 h of sitting, as well as reaching the physical activity recommendation may help counteract the potential negative effect of too much sitting time. Governments must provide active free time options to promote active leisure time and help reduce screen time. At workplaces, managers and companies should encourage sitting breaks and work standing options, and for the special population such as children or older adults, new strategies must be considered to reduce sitting time.

Keywords: sitting time, exercise, older adults, children, work time, leisure time, sedentary breaks

1. Introduction

Lifestyle has changed over the world in the past decades. The industrialization process and technological advances have simplified the physical work of human beings and changed the lifestyle of the last generations. Not that long ago, most of the jobs required physical activity and some energy expenditure. Nowadays the percentage of work sectors demanding high levels of physical activity has reduced drastically. This new reality derives in many people forced to spend at more than 8 h/day sitting and having difficulties to reach the physical activity recommendations [1]. Sedentary lifestyles have become a significant public health issue spreading worldwide, although there is evidence of being linked to a range of chronic health conditions [2]. Extended periods of inactivity can produce metabolic dysfunction and impair blood sugar regulation [3], elevate blood pressure [4], and make it difficult to use fat as a metabolic substrate, as well as increase the risk of early death regardless of physical activity levels [5]. Therefore, it seems crucial to find strategies that can be applied in all life domains to be able to reduce sedentary behavior, as well as to increase physical activity. Including regular and well-structured sedentary breaks during long sitting periods could help reduce the negative effects of a sedentary lifestyle.

This chapter aimed, firstly, to provide scientific evidence of the need to reduce sedentary behaviors as well as to include regularly sedentary breaks. Secondly, to show some possibilities and examples of how to break sedentarism in daily life. We believe that introducing these practices in workspaces, schools, leisure time, and in the daily activities of older adults might help control the negative effects derived from sedentary lifestyles.

2. Sedentary behavior

2.1 Evolution of lifestyle and the concept of sedentary behavior

Historically, exercise physiologists have studied sedentary lifestyle as the opposite of physical activity. The terms that have been used for research in this area have been confusing, which makes it difficult to compare clinical trials. Already in the 1950s, Morris et al. [6] concluded that sedentary work increased cardiovascular risk compared to those who worked more physically active. That study, among others, resulted in a strong area of research focused, for over 60 years, on quantifying the level of physical activity necessary to reduce morbidity and mortality [6]. These investigations provided recommendations on physical activity and the implementation of public policies to promote physical activity practice.

Despite the efforts, a high percentage of the population (mostly from countries that suffered rapid urbanization and industrialization) do no reach the physical activity recommendations and the tendency is that this number increases [1] Office works, school, screen games, technology, passive transportation and sedentary leisure time have had a strong impact on reducing the opportunities to perform physical activity at the same time that promote opportunities for sedentary behavior in all the life domains.

For the past two decades, the number of studies focused on sedentary behavior has grown exponentially, and physical activity and sedentary behavior can be considered as an independent research field. The term sedentary behavior comes from Latin "sedere" which means "to sit". But not only the "position" determines what is currently conceived as sedentary behavior. Sedentary behavior is defined as any waking behavior characterized by the expenditure of 1.5 metabolic equivalents of task (MET)s or less of energy while in a sitting, reclining, or lying posture [7]. Sedentary behavior, like physical activity, can be found in all life domains (work, study, transport, and free time). Although research in this field has increased notably in the last decade, there is still confusion in the terminology and the scientific community has not reached a consensus in some terms and concepts yet. Many definitions of sedentary behavior can be found in the literature but some common concepts are repeated, such as low energy expenditure, mostly under 1.5 METs, activities performed in sitting, lying or reclining position and while the person is awake [7]. Besides, some other concepts associated with sedentary behavior have aroused the interest of the scientific community. Sedentary bouts, breaks of sitting, sedentarism, sedentary lifestyle vs. inactivity, among others, are related terms that could help deeply understand this problem.

Sedentary Behavior Concept has suffer an evolution over the years. Although the distinction between sedentarism and physical inactivity (not meeting worldwide recommendations for physical activity) has already been settled [7], it is still common to find some confusion in terms such as sedentary time, sitting time, screen time and stationary time; which, although in some cases are overlapping concepts, refer to different behaviors [7]. Because they refer to different aspects of behavior (position, movement, effort and the use of digital implements), these traits can be blended in different ways, so that some criteria are met but others are not. For example, one can be seated but doing physical activity (cycloergometer), so it's not a sedentary behavior; one could be stationary, but not sitting (e.g., waiting in line); one may be in sedentary behavior, but not sitting (instead lying down watching TV), which in turn is independent of screen usage (reading a book); among other examples.

2.2 Using bed rest models

Studies on bed rest [8–13] provided useful information on the consequences of inactivity and low energy expenditure for long periods. Thanks to these studies, a lot is known about the effects of prolonged inactivity in metabolism and organ systems. Different studies focused on the effects of bed rest on metabolic function, found peripheral insulin resistance in skeletal muscle and adipose tissue, hepatic insulin resistance and a dyslipidemia [10], as well as a decline in function, muscle mass, and muscle strength [12] and a reduction in cardiorespiratory capacity after one-week bed rest [13]. In regards to the musculoskeletal structure, inactivity produces loss of strength and endurance, contractures, changes in soft tissues, disuse osteoporosis, sarcopenia, and degenerative joint disease [8]. At the cardiovascular level, the consequences can be postural hypotension, cardiac dysfunction, and thrombotic events [13]. Additionally, bed rest can lead to impaired respiratory, renal, gastrointestinal, and nervous system levels [9]. Outside hospitalization or illness, free-living healthy adults rarely spend these amounts of bed rest. Nevertheless, technological and social factors have made prolonged sitting time a common practice in all life domains (work, domestic life, and leisure time).

2.3 Quantifying sedentary behavior

Measuring physical activity and sitting time is complex. Research has been aimed at improving the quality of the data through the objective measurement of sedentary behavior using accelerometry, observing that the self-report measurement underestimates the daily time of sedentary behavior concerning the objective measurement.

Researchers have focused on developing devices to be able to objectively quantify physical activity. In the past decades, many studies using accelerometers have been carried out. A multi-country study (USA, Brazil, UK, Denmark, the Czech Republic, and Hong Kong) using accelerometry found that the average sedentary time per day was 513 min/day, or 8.55 h/day [14]. Sedentary time was estimated to be responsible for 3.8% of all-cause mortality in adults according to a meta-analysis pooling data across 54 countries [15]. The United States Physical Activity Guidelines Advisory Committee (PAGAC) [16] recently comprehensively reviewed the scientific evidence, linking sedentary behavior with specific physical health indicators in adults and older adults, including mortality, cardiovascular disease, type 2 diabetes, cancer, and obesity. Moreover, high levels of sedentary behavior are also negative associated with cognitive function, depression, function and disability, physical activity levels, and health-related quality of life [17]. In contrast, little evidence has demonstrated the relationship between sedentary behavior and musculoskeletal pain, accidents or injuries, fatigue, sleep, or work productivity [18]. Ku et al. [19] published in 2018 a meta-regression analysis involving more than 1 million participants in which the cut-off points of daily sedentary time that were related to all-cause mortality in adults were established for data measured objectively and self-reported [19]. According to the results of the study, the method of measuring sitting time significantly moderated the association between daily sitting time and mortality risk. The cut-off of daily sitting time in studies with self-report data was 7 h/day in comparison with 9 h/day for those with data measured by devices.

2.4 Sedentary behavior VS physical activity

It is accepted that exercise is an effective strategy for reducing key cardiovascular risks [20]. Nevertheless, it is unclear if the benefits can be modified by a sedentary lifestyle. Therefore, it is important to clearly define different concepts such as physical activity/inactivity or sedentary behavior, as their physiological consequences on health are different. While physical activity/inactivity is referred to whether or not a person reaches the physical activity recommendations, a person is considered as sedentary if he/she spends long periods of the day in sedentary behavior. While for the first one (cut-off points for being physically active) there is enough evidence to determine the recommendations (150 minutes of moderate physical activity or 75 minutes of vigorous physical activity or an equivalent metabolic combination between both, plus 2–3 days/week of resistance training) [21], for the second one (cut-off points for being sedentary) there are still no recommendations, since studies have found inconclusive results.

That means that a person can meet the physical activity guidelines and still be considered sedentary. Sedentary behavior might produce harmful effects on health independently of physical activity level, but when both are combined, the results seem to change (combined joint association). In other words, high levels of sedentary behavior combined with low levels of physical activity increase the risk of death by 46% [18]. On the contrary, some studies have shown that high levels of physical activity can counteract or reduce the risk of death caused by prolonged sedentary behavior [22]. Similar results were obtained in cancer patients, where in the most active patients no relationship was observed between sedentary behavior and cancer mortality, while for those less active the risk of death increased [23].

Using the concepts of sedentary and/or physically active person, we can describe four possible combinations:

A. **The sedentary inactive:** Those who do not meet the physical activity recommendations and also spend long periods of the day sitting.

B. **The non-sedentary inactive:** Those who do not meet the physical activity recommendations but do not spend long periods of the day sitting.

C. **The sedentary active:** Those who reach the physical activity recommendation but spend long periods of the day sitting.

D. **The non-sedentary active:** Those who reach the physical activity recommendations and also do not spend long periods of the day sitting.

Figure 1 represents graphically these possibilities.

The health implication for possibilities A and D are clear. Classification A has a negative influence on health and is negatively associated with all-cause mortality and D is positively associated with better health markers. What is not fully clear yet, are the implications of classifications B and C. Can one the variables counteract the negative effect of too much of the other one? Or, are the positive effects of one variable suppressed by the other one?

CLASSIFICATION	SEDENTARY	NON SEDENTARY
NOT PHYSICALLY ACTIVE	A. Not reaching the PA recommendations AND sitting for long periods X	B. Not reaching the PA recommendations BUT not sitting for long periods ?
PHYSICALLY ACTIVE	C. Reaching the PA recommendations BUT sitting for long periods ?	D. Reaching the PA recommendations AND is not sitting for long periods ✓

Figure 1.
Person's classification according to sedentary behavior and physical activity practice. (A) Sedentary inactive, (B) non-sedentay inactive, (C) sedentary active, (D) non-sedentary active.

As mentioned before, some studies found that high levels of physical activity might attenuate the increased risk of some illness or death associated with high sitting times [22]. Notwithstanding, there is still some uncertainty in the characteristics of the specific dose–response curves, which makes it difficult to determine specific quantitative public health recommendations [24]. As sedentary lifestyle in western societies does not tend to reduce, new strategies might be the solution. Some degree of sedentary lifestyle might be beneficial for health so that it helps to rest and recover. On the contrary, excessive sitting time may become a risk factor. Scientific evidence has not found an increase in the risk of death from any cause in people with a total sitting time between 4–8 hours/day when compared to those who remain seated for less than 4 hours. Nevertheless, the risk increases by 15% when sitting time rises to 8–11 hours/day, and by 40% with sitting times higher than 11 hours/day [25]. Contrary, some other studies found a dose–response relationship for every 1-hour increase in sitting time in intervals between 0–3, >3–7, and > 7 h/day total sitting and all-cause mortality. This model estimated a 34% higher mortality risk for adults sitting 10 h/day, after taking physical activity into account, although the risk increased staggered [26], similar to other studies that observed statistically significantly higher risk of death with sedentary times of 9.5 h/day or more [23].

This situation has put the focus on the double challenge of increasing levels of physical activity and reducing sedentary behavior. Many countries have developed strategies to promote changes in the population. As an example, the Canadian government created the Canadian 24-Hour Movement Guidelines for Adults (https://csepguidelines.ca/). It recommends that adults between 18–64 years must limit sedentary time to 8 hours/day or less, including no more than 3 hours/day of recreation screen time and breaking long periods of sitting as often as possible.

2.5 Sedentary breaks: effectivity of the different types according to scientific evidence

As it has been mentioned before, modern lifestyles predispose a high percentage of the population to spend long periods in sedentary behaviors. As too much sitting time is related to different chronic diseases such as type 2 diabetes, obesity, hypertension, and cardiovascular diseases, or some types of cancer, it seems crucial to clearly understand the mechanism and strategies to reduce the negative effects of a sedentary lifestyle. Generalizing, we get up, use the elevator to go to the car, drive to work, take the escalator to go work, spend 8 hours at least working with minimum movement, drive back home, eat, have some hours of recreational time, watch TV and go to bed. Fortunately, different lifestyles and personal situations (occupational situation and leisure-time preferences) as well as inherent individual differences, result in different accumulations of sedentary time. Due to the strong available evidence on the deleterious effects of a sedentary lifestyle on health, it is necessary to better understand the metabolic mechanisms and how it is accumulated. Researchers have observed that reducing or breaking up sedentary time may result in beneficial changes in body composition and acute improvements in markers of cardiometabolic risk.

Sedentary behavior might be considered as a multifactorial concept, where four different aspects influencing it should be taken into account:

a. **Type of activity performed seated:** intellectual or occupational sitting seems to be less harmful than TV time or less intellectual activities.

b. **Level of PA:** adequate levels of physical activity may attenuate the negative effect of prolonged sitting.

c. **Age:** as an accumulative factor, so that, normally, if a person has a sedentary lifestyle, it has been adopted for more years when the person is older and the deleterious effects have been applying longer.

d. **Interruptions in sedentary bouts**: interrupting sitting time regularly may attenuate its negative effects when comparing to the same average uninterrupted sitting time.

It has been proposed that breaks in sedentary time could help counteract the negative effect of prolonged periods of whole-body inactivity. A break in sedentary time can be defined as a period of non-sedentary activity, such as standing or walking in between two sedentary bouts [7]. Experimental studies have demonstrated that interrupting sedentary time with short frequent breaks reduces daily glucose, postprandial glucose, and insulin resistance [3, 26, 27]. In a study carried out by Healy et al. [28] in 2008, the authors found, that interruptions of sedentary behavior were negatively associated with obesity and cardiometabolic health. These results highlighted, already at that time, the fact that not only total sitting matters but also how it is distributed in a period of time. The characteristic of the sedentary breaks in the study from Healy et al. showed that the breaks reported by the participants were shorter than 5 min on average, and they were performed at a light intensity. Results from this study also found lower waist circumference, BMI, triglycerides, and 2-h plasma glucose in the participants with higher sedentary break bouts, independent of total sedentary time or moderate-to-vigorous intensity activity time. Since this pioneering study was published, the scientific community have had an increased interest in analyzing the effects of sedentary breaks, to be able to deeply understand the effects of prolonged sitting on metabolism, as well as to establish clear and specific guidelines of intervention. Different types of sedentary breaks have been studied trying to analyze if shorter bouts of sitting time, are less metabolic disrupting even when the total amount of daily or weekly sitting times are similar.

Brief bouts of light-intensity-activity sedentary breaks could reduce the negative effects of long periods sitting on lower limb vascular function in healthy and overweight/obese adults [29]. Experimental studies [30–32] have seen that combining exercise with breaks in sitting resulted in additional reductions in postprandial insulin-glucose dynamics and triglycerides when comparing exercise and uninterrupted sitting. This effect, although useful in any case, seems to be more effective in those with high basal insulin resistance.

As many studies focused on analyzing the effects of sedentary breaks to counteract the metabolic problems associated with prolonged sitting time have found positive interactions, the question that remains unanswered is not if we should break sitting regularly, what already has a positive answer. The unanswered question is, which is the best structure for a sedentary break?

As it has been mentioned before, the lack of enough specific interventional studies complicates for experts to concrete the most optimal structure for sedentary breaks. A recent study by Wheeler et al. [30] investigated the effects of 3 different sitting strategies in overweight and obese: i) uninterrupted sitting for 8 h, ii) sitting for 1 h, moderate-intensity walking for 30-min and uninterrupted sitting for 6.5 h and iii) sitting for 1 h, moderate-intensity walking for 30 min and sitting for 6.5 h interrupting sitting every 30 min with 3 min of light-intensity walking. They found reductions in postprandial insulin-glucose dynamics and triglycerides by combining exercise with breaks in sitting. This study not only proposes a way to help reach the physical activity recommendation by breaking sedentary time for 30 min/day but also demonstrates that regular sedentary breaks help control the metabolic deleterious effect of prolonged sitting.

A well-controlled meta-analysis conducted by Loh et al. in 2020 [33] found that the use of sitting breaks moderately attenuated post-prandial glucose, insulin, and triacylglycerol. The authors also found that the glycemic attenuation was greater in people with a higher body mass index. An interesting result was that for attenuating glucose levels, a statistically significant small advantage for sitting breaks was found over continuous exercise when exercise matched energy. That could mean that for glucose regulation, it might be more interesting short regular breaks along the day, than one continuous bout of exercise.

The skeletal muscle might also play a key role in glycaemia control, which is even more important in overweight. Bergouignan et al. [34] performed an analysis from randomized clinical trials comparing one or three days uninterrupted sitting with sitting interrupted with light-intensity or moderate-intensity walking every 20-min in the modulation of contraction- and insulin-stimulated glucose uptake pathways in muscle. They found that both sitting break interventions reduced postprandial glucose concentration as well as a transition to modulation of the insulin-signaling pathway and increased capacity for glucose transport. The moderate-intensity intervention resulted in a greater capacity for glycogen synthesis and ATP production. These results might through some light in preventive strategy for metabolic diseases.

Published literature [35] might tend to propose that the best option to reduce the negative effects of sedentary behavior on metabolic functions could be to combine regular activity breaks of several minutes every 30 min of sitting with 30 min of continuous walking whether at the beginning or the end of the long sitting period.

Therefore, breaking sedentary time should be a good way to reduce the negative effects of long periods of sitting, for both metabolic and muscle function. These breaks are even more interesting for patients with initial high blood sugar, insulin resistance, or overweight-obesity. The general recommendation would be to make an active 2–3 min-break every 30 min of sitting time. If the activity made during these breaks is of moderate-high intensity, such as climbing stairs, the metabolic benefits might be greater.

2.6 Sedentary behavior in the workplace. Strategies

The workplace is considered an important environment for the promotion and protection of health [36]. According to a report from the World Health Organization (WHO) together with the World Economic Forum, 65% of the world's adult population is part of the workforce [37]. In 2007, about 3.1 billion people were part of the economically active population and it was estimated that by 2021 this number would exceed 3.6 billion [38]. Taking into account that this working adult population spends around a third of the day at work, workers´ health must be seen as a priority action.

Encouraging the reduction of sedentary behavior and promoting the practice of physical activity in the workplace is a strategy that helps maintain the health of the working population and affects their close environment. In 2018, the WHO presented the Global Action Plan for Physical Activity [39], with two mean challenges: reducing sedentary behavior by 2030 as well as the percentage of inactive population by 15% to the reported values of 2016. This plan encourages the population to take advantage of the many opportunities that arise in daily living to integrate physical activity, including the workplace (as a fundamental environment to practice physical activity programs as well as its promotion).

The activities where sedentary behavior predominates have increased lately and the workplace is a clear example. The machines have replaced human physical work at the same time that there has been a notable increase in office jobs, where the employee spends most of the working day in front of a computer. Although the negative consequences for cardiometabolic and musculoskeletal health of sedentary behavior have been widely demonstrated and office work represents for many workers a third of their day sitting, few have been made to improve this situation and reduce sitting time at workplaces, with the associated health risk.

The Healthy Work Environment model, proposed by the WHO [38] proposes intervention programs to reduce and break sedentary behavior in the workplace as a health promotion model and protection strategy. This model proposes four scenarios of action or "avenues of influence", which are not isolated, but rather overlap each other:

1. The physical environment of the work, which refers to the structure, air, machinery, furniture.

2. The psychosocial work environment, which includes the organization of work and institutional culture, attitudes, values, beliefs that can affect the mental and physical well-being of workers.

3. Personal health resources in the workplace, that consist in an environment that promotes health, health services, information, resources, opportunities, and the flexibility that the companies offer to workers to support the efforts to improve or maintain healthy lifestyles, as well as to monitor and support your physical and mental health.

4. The physical participation of the institution in the community, which includes the activities that the company carries out to improve the safety, well-being, and quality of life of workers and their families.

To successfully establish health promotion programs in the workplace, certain conditions must be considered:

1. Raising awareness among managers and chiefs of the importance of these interventions, facilitating employees to carry them out. Companies' leaders must understand that these strategies are not only not time wasted but will also result in increased productivity.

2. A previous evaluation of the workplace and the type of tasks that are developed, that help design an optimal plan.

3. Execution of the plan with the support of all interested parts (managers, middle managers, bosses, CEO, etc.) and commitment by workers.

4. Re-evaluation and adaptation of the proposal.

With different adaptations, similar models can be recommended with more or less the same stages.

Experts have suggested different strategies to reduce or interrupt sedentary behavior in the workplace, which could be grouped into the following categories [40].

a. Physical/environmental changes in workplace design

- Desks with adjustable height that allow lifting them to work standing up.

- Raised desks with a treadmill.

- Rooms with high tables for standing meetings.

- Modify the layout of the workplace, for example, by placing printers, trashcans, or water dispensers away from desks, which will force employees to stand up and walk a few steps when they need to use these items.

- Provide bicycle racks, lockers, and services to wash up to encourage active transportation to work.

- Eliminate architectural barriers to allow employees to move around the workplace, creating unobstructed corridors and spaces that invite walking.

b. Changes in workplace policy to incentivize and encourage reduction and disruption of sitting time

- Promote the holding of standing or walking meetings.

- Propose active breaks during working hours (short breaks in which you can do joint mobility exercises, put on a musical theme and dance, or any activity that allows interrupting the sedentary behavior through light physical activity)

- Offer group physical activity practice.

- Encourage the use of breaks for short walks.

- Encourage employees to communicate with their colleagues by approaching their desks rather than by phone or messages.

- Propose to take advantage of telephone communications to do them standing or walking (obviously, spaces that do not interfere with the work of others should be considered).

- Encourage the use of the stairs instead of the elevator or escalator.

c. Information and advice to raise employee awareness and commitment by offering

- Workshops, training courses and outreach programs on the importance of reducing sedentary behavior. Reporting on the health risks of sedentary behavior and the benefits of practicing physical activity could allow people to evaluate their behavioral choices.

- Campaigns through various means, such as posters, signage, emails, WhatsApp messages, telephone calls or internal messages to motivate a change in behavior or.

- Install reminder software every 30 minutes on employees' mobile phones or personal computers, for example, to interrupt the sedentary behavior by standing up, dancing or doing some movements.

2.7 Sedentary behavior in the leisure time. Strategies

As mentioned so far, human bodies are adapted to maintain a physically active lifestyle. Proof of this is the health consequences of an insufficient level of physical activity. However, it is also true that neurobiologically we are adapted to "optimize" our energy expenditure, avoiding additional efforts when possible; In other words, sedentary behaviors are attractive for human beings, and willing power is required to counteract this attraction and opt for a behavior with higher associated energy expenditure [41]. It has been studied how the energy cost associated with a task affects, not only our decision to choose another more "economic" one, but directly to our perception of the initial task [42] and, therefore, to our future intention to undertake it.

A process as complex as human behavior cannot be reduced to just one component. Emotional/affective factors, as well as built habits, are also related to sedentary behavior and physical activity [43]. However, it is an interesting starting point if we seek an alternative approach to the one traditionally used. The assumption that human behaviors are decided by rational evaluations of the available information are underlying concepts in many current intervention strategies and, therefore, knowing the benefits of regular physical activity and the damages of prolonged sedentary behavior should be enough to solve the problem [44]. Nevertheless, in light of the sustained global pandemic of physical inactivity, it may be necessary to complement and enrich this approach with other perspectives.

Sedentary behaviors in free time are usually classified as screen-time (watching television, videos via streaming platform or physical medium, browsing the internet and social networks by both on a computer, tablet or cell phone and the use of video games) or not screen-time (sitting down to eat, participating in social gatherings, playing board games, recreational, attending cultural events such as cinema, theater, show music, sports competition, religious ceremony, doing artistic activities like writing or drawing or hobbies. The extensive list is testimony to the enormous offer of sedentary activities in free time. Recommendations on physical activity and sedentary behavior limit the amount of time in sedentary behaviors, but particularly those carried out in front of the screen [21].

Sedentary activities in front of the screen in free time, in addition to adverse effects on physical health, are related to adverse effects on mental health, mainly in minors [45]. Screen time during childhood is negatively correlated with brain connectivity, compared to time spent reading books, as well as being related to loss of imagery ability [46] or social–emotional functionality [47]. Interestingly, and in contrast to these studies, in the specific case of video games, there is evidence that indicates various cognitive benefits according to the type of game (action, strategy), and even positive socio-emotional impacts [48].

Of the large number of sedentary activities carried out in free time, although the impact on physical health is equivalent, it would be differential over other dimensions of the subject's health. This leads to one of the perspectives mentioned in the literature as a strategy to address sedentary behavior: "harm reduction". Assuming that certain socio-cultural (technological) changes are already part of daily life, priority is given to modifying those behaviors that present a greater health risk: replacing sedentary behaviors in front of the screen with sedentary behaviors without a screen, or by non-sedentary screen activities (for example, walking while using portable devices or replacing sedentary video games with active ones) [49].

Different classifications have been proposed for reducing sedentary behavior in the free time [50]: 1) environmental interventions such as devices that limit the time of television use), and 2) behavioral interventions like education campaigns about the harms of prolonged sedentary behavior; 3) multi-component interventions which include both types mentioned above.

Although studies on this fact do not have homogeneous methodologies, some findings can be pointed out. Studies that focus on the sedentary behavior of children in the home context have found a relationship between the existence of screen devices in the bedroom and greater sedentary behavior (with less reading time). Likewise, both the interventions that use devices that limit the use of television and those on family rules for screen use have been successful in reducing sedentary behavior. Furthermore, it was observed that in those cases in which the parents had more television time, or participated with their children in sedentary activities, the children presented higher levels of sedentary behavior. In some studies, the existence of adequate space or equipment for practicing physical activity at home is related to less sedentary behavior (although it does not present higher levels of physical activity at moderate or vigorous intensities) [51].

In the case of adults and the elderly, studies on free time are scarce and methodological imprecise. The absence of control in the domains makes it difficult to control the changes since the decrease of sedentary time in a domain does not imply its replacement by physical activity since it could simply shift to sedentary behavior in another domain. Those interventions aimed exclusively at reducing sedentary behavior have better results than those that also focused on increasing physical activity [50].

For children and adolescents, as well as for adults and the elderly, there is another alternative intervention strategy, which constitutes itself in an emerging field of research: exergaming, also known as active gaming or effort video game. These video games, unlike the traditional ones, are controlled with body movements (either full body or only certain segments); Thus, instead of being a sedentary activity, at least light-intensity physical activity is achieved (with the potential to become moderate intensity and even vigorous). In the US, it is estimated that 90% of children and adolescents play video games recreationally. In an increasing technophile society, and in which electronic entertainment is already part of our lives, exergaming stands as a strategy to address those to whom other physical activity proposals are not convincing. In addition, the commitment, immersion, and experience of "flow" that they can generate, make them a great resource for health-related purposes. Sustainability over the years of this type of activity has been investigated, finding greater adherence in women, and similar to that of team sports [52].

Results for studies analyzing experiences in exergaming as part of both school physical education and at-home context show a decrease in sedentary behavior with potential, according to the intensity at which the game is played, increase of moderate-to-vigorous physical activity and good adherence to intervention programs. One of the challenges of exergaming is the "replay value" (once the game becomes monotonous and therefore the motivation to continue playing decreases), which maintain adherence. Multiplayer games (both face-to-face and remotely) show greater adherence. The eventual increase in the number of published games would compensate for this situation, allowing simply to change to a new one [53].

Particularly interesting is the research with older people, which improvements for both institutionalized and community-dwelling subjects, and not only in the physical dimensions but also in the cognitive one [54].

In all these cases, we refer mainly to consoles-home exergaming, but everyday mobile devices with augmented reality technology (Pokémon Go with geo-location system integrated into cell phones) are great opportunities to promote exergaming. Pokémon Go requires active movement of the player around their surroundings to play. This game mechanic has achieved a statistically significant change in the number of steps per day (thus decreasing sedentary behavior), although there is still not enough evidence on long-term adherence.

In the latter case, as in some home exergaming video games, there is no explicit intention in its design to promote health effects or to prescribe a systematic physical activity program. However, they have the potential to have a positive impact on the health and well-being of those who opt for this type of digital entertainment. Sedentary behavior in free time poses a great global challenge that requires, particularly for new generations, imagination and innovative approaches, in tune with contemporary technologies and paradigms.

2.8 Sedentary behavior in special populations: children and adolescents and older people. Strategies

2.8.1 Children and adolescents

It is well accepted that physical activity is beneficial to maintain and improve health and well-being across life [55]. In infants, toddlers, and preschoolers, high levels of physical activity have been seen to be related to better social and motor development improved metabolic health, and decreased adiposity, while a sedentary lifestyle is related to higher adiposity and poorer psychosocial health and cognitive development [54].

Children (preschoolers and scholars) spend more than 2 h/day of screen time, which is the maximal time recommended for this age group [56], plus eating time, school, passive transportation, homework, etc., which results in more than 8 h/day of sitting at this age. Moreover, studies found that screen time was associated with an increased risk of overweight/obese independent of physical activity [54]. Sex differences were also found. Boys are generally more involved in physical activity than girls, which normally spent more time on domestic tasks and homework. Children living in rural areas tend to use more active transportation than those who live in urban areas. Older children also tend to use more active transportation than the younger ones [57]. Taking into account that sedentary behavior in children is directly associated with classical cardiovascular risk factors like elevated blood glucose levels, insulin resistance, high blood pressure, obesity, and elevated blood lipids [58], strategies that help reduce total daily sitting time in children are crucial.

Nevertheless, although childhood should be a life stage where children should freely play, run and jump as part of their natural development, social rules, obligations, parent's overprotection, new technologies, and urban environments, hinder the practice of physical activity for children with dramatic consequences. A qualitative study performed by Hidding et al. [59] aimed in determining the reasons for children to be sitting from the children or parents perspective, found that children most repeated reason was that they sit because is the norm and they have to and because they can play better that way. Other common answers were: I sit because seated activities are fun, I sit because I'm tired, I want to relax, I want to rest, I sit because of my health, I sit because there is nobody to play with, I sit because there is nothing to do, I sit because I'm not in the mood to do anything, I sit because of the weather. In regards to the answer "I sit because there is nobody to play with", in families with more than one child, seems to be easy for children to perform physical activity [59].

All this information brings the experts 'awareness of the necessity of reconsider children's environments. The CSEP Canadian 24-Hour Movement Guidelines [56] propose an Integration of physical activity (both light and moderate-to-vigorous), sedentary behavior, and sleep as the three principal parts of the day. All three must be right balanced to promote overall health, well-being, and quality of life. These guidelines use "the four S rule":

1. SWEAT: Moderate to Vigorous Physical Activity: An accumulation of at least 60 min/day.

2. STEP: Light physical activity: Several hours of a variety of structured and unstructured light physical activities (playing, walking)

3. SLEEP: Uninterrupted 9 to 11 h/night for those aged 5–13 years and 8 to 10 h/night for those aged 14–17 years, with consistent bed and wake-up times.

4. SIT: Sedentary behavior: No more than 2 h/day of recreational screen time and limited sitting for extended periods.

Figure 2 ilustrates de cited guidelines.

In addition, parents might consider changing indoor activities for outdoor ones, when possible, and including moderate to vigorous physical activity in exchange for light physical activity at some point of the day.

Findings from a recent meta-analysis [60] on the physical activity a sedentary behavior suggest that physical activity interventions can improve adolescents' mental health.

2.8.2 Older adults

Worldwide, the population is aging, which results in higher economic and social costs, as well as increased numbers of people living with more health problems, as aging increases the risk of suffering from chronic diseases. Therefore, the concept of successful aging has become a priority to guarantee, not only that life expectancy is high, but also that the years lived are of the best quality possible, free or with minimum chronic diseases. Physical activity has been proven to help increase or maintain health throughout life. Due to physical activity tends to reduce with age, older adults must become a risk population. Disability, frailty, dysfunction,

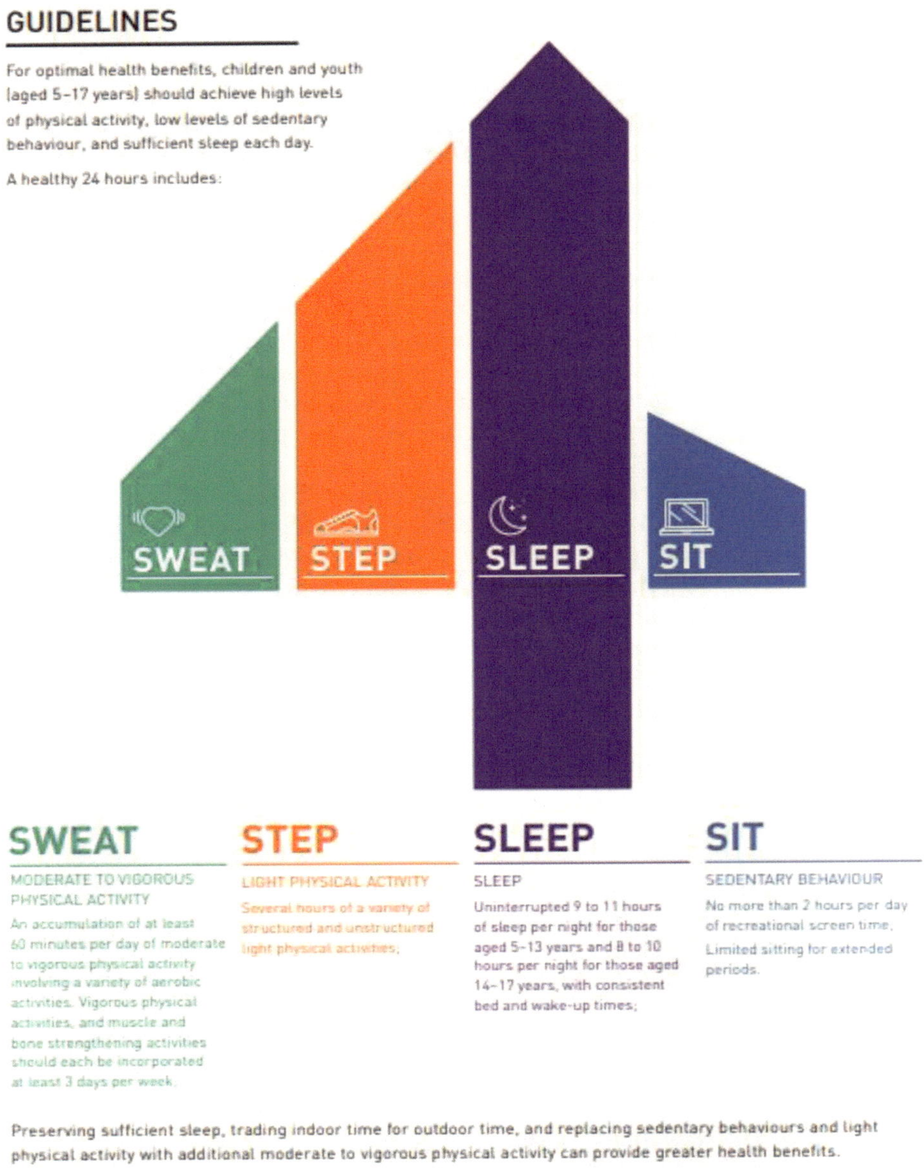
GUIDELINES
For optimal health benefits, children and youth (aged 5-17 years) should achieve high levels of physical activity, low levels of sedentary behaviour, and sufficient sleep each day.
A healthy 24 hours includes:
SWEAT
STEP
SLEEP
SIT
SWEAT
MODERATE TO VIGOROUS PHYSICAL ACTIVITY
An accumulation of at least 60 minutes per day of moderate to vigorous physical activity involving a variety of aerobic activities. Vigorous physical activities, and muscle and bone strengthening activities should each be incorporated at least 3 days per week;
STEP
LIGHT PHYSICAL ACTIVITY
Several hours of a variety of structured and unstructured light physical activities;
SLEEP
SLEEP
Uninterrupted 9 to 11 hours of sleep per night for those aged 5-13 years and 8 to 10 hours per night for those aged 14-17 years, with consistent bed and wake-up times;
SIT
SEDENTARY BEHAVIOUR
No more than 2 hours per day of recreational screen time;
Limited sitting for extended periods.
Preserving sufficient sleep, trading indoor time for outdoor time, and replacing sedentary behaviours and light physical activity with additional moderate to vigorous physical activity can provide greater health benefits.

Figure 2.
Canadian 24-hour movement guidelines for children and youth (5-17 years): an integration of physical activity, sedentary behavior, and sleep. Taken from CSEP website (https://csepguidelines.ca/).

or sarcopenia are some of the problems that can affect older adults, which can compromise the independence level [61]. As physical activity decreases in this group, sedentary behavior increases, with fatal consequences. Maintaining physical activity levels and reducing sedentary time, should be a priority for the administrations. In this regard, there is evidence about the negative associations of sedentary behavior with frailty and how this relationship can differ by sitting bout length. Some studies [62] have found that prolonged sedentary bouts and total sedentary time were associated with higher mortality risk in frail individuals but not in robust. These results, including moderate-to-vigorous physical activity, reducing sedentary time in those frail older adults, as well as including sedentary breaks seem like a suitable strategy to prevent dependency and maintain health. As the total hours of a day are always 24, that means that when a person increases the time spent in moderate-to-vigorous physical activity, this person is reducing the time spent in another activity, that could be sitting or light physical activity. If sleeping time remains stable and a person substitutes 30 min/day of light physical activity for moderate-to-vigorous physical activity that includes resistance training, and at the same time changes 1 hour of sitting for light physical activity such as walking, the frailty status could be significantly reduced. Moreover, if this person would include a short sedentary break every 30 min - 1 hour of the total time this person is seated, the benefits would be even higher with only small changes.

Due to older adults are mostly retired, which releases them of office sitting time and have a lot of leisure time, political strategies must center on providing older adults with a safe environment where they can perform light physical activity, such as walking [63]. Pavements and sidewalks in good conditions, green areas, and safe cross-roads might help improve that older adults go more often outside to take a walk. At the same time, organized affordable exercise activities, specifically designed by experts for this population, could make that older adult reach the recommendation for moderate-to-vigorous physical activity and resistance training. Moreover, these activities also promote social interaction, which improve wellbeing and might help reduce depression and anxiety, improving health-related quality of life, as well. These two actions would help to achieve physical activity recommendations at the same time that sedentary time would be reduced. To completely promote health in this group, clinicians, governments, and media should establish campaigns to make older adults understand the importance of breaking sedentary time. Things such as get up in the commercials when they watch TV, walking or standing while they are phoning, or get up to drink some water once each hour might be enough to break sitting time.

3. Conclusions

Lifestyle has dramatically changed in the last century. Industrialization and technology have reduced the physical requirements of many jobs, urbanization has changed population habits, force them to use passive transport instead of active ones, children play with digital devices since they are very young and older adult do not have to go outside because cities, family and environment easily provide all their needs. However, this sedentary lifestyle has disastrous consequences for health. Physical activity is necessary to maintain an optimal physiological function and prolonged sitting time interferes with the proper metabolic regulation. The combination of both, low physical activity levels and prolonged sitting time, maybe even more deleterious. That suggests a double challenge for developed countries; reducing and stopping prolonged sedentary behavior as well as increasing levels of physical activity. Although each of them separately has concrete effects on health, their interaction must be also taken into account. Sedentary behavior appears to be negative for health "per se", as well as low physical activity levels, but how both are combined is what can make the difference. Scientific evidence says that high physical activity levels might help counteract the negative effects of sitting time and that this effect is progressive. That means, that the higher the physical activity intensity, the less negative effects of sitting time. At the same time, it seems that long continuous sitting bouts are more harmful than the same total sitting time but with breaks in between. Eight hours seated without any break might be a lot worse for metabolic regulation than the same 8 h of sitting but with breaks of 2–3 min every 30 min-1 h. With all these ideas in mind, the strategy to reduce sedentary behavior seems clear: practice enough physical activity, reduce free-time sitting and screen time, promote active transportation, and include sedentary breaks at sedentary jobs. The reason why these strategies are not working is complex and implies a compromise at different levels. First, governments must provide opportunities for affordable exercise practice and physical activity-friendly environments. Secondly, at workplaces, managers, CEOs, and bosses must be aware of the importance of promoting working places where employees have the opportunity of breaking sedentary time, and that it is seen as normal. Third, citizens should make efforts to include active activities in the free time as well as substitute classic videogames for exergaming, where at least, sitting time is exchanged for light physical activity. Last but not least, special populations (children and older adults) should not be forgotten. Parents and schools should reconsider the rules and norms and adapt them, when possible, to others more active versions, not forcing children to spend long periods seated promoting at the same time at least one hour of physical activity per day. Controlling screen time and giving good examples must be another priority for parents. In regards to older adults, societies should allow them to perform easy tasks that increase physical activity, encouraging them to used active transportations to carry them out, at the same time that exercise programs, specifical design for this population, are easily available in every neighborhood.

Author details

Olga López Torres[1*], Pablo Lobo[2], Valeria Baigún[2] and Gabriela F. De Roia[2]

1 ImFINE Research Group, Health and Human Performance Department, Faculty of Physical Activity and Port Science-INEF, Universidad Politécnica de Madrid, Madrid, Spain

2 Laboratorio de Estudios en Actividad Física, Universidad de Flores, Ciudad Autónoma de Buenos Aires, Argentina

*Address all correspondence to: olga.lopez@upm.es

References

[1] Guthold R, Stevens GA, Riley LM, Bull FC. Worldwide trends in insufficient physical activity from 2001 to 2016: a pooled analysis of 358 population-based surveys with 1·9 million participants. Lancet Glob Heal [Internet]. 2018;6(10):e1077-86. Available from: http://dx.doi.org/10.1016/S2214-109X(18)30357-7

[2] Chau JY, Grunseit AC, Chey T, Stamatakis E, Brown WJ, Matthews CE, et al. Daily sitting time and all-cause mortality: A meta-analysis. PLoS One. 2013;8(11):1-14.

[3] Chastin SFM, Egerton T, Leask C, Stamatakis E. Meta-analysis of the relationship between breaks in sedentary behavior and cardiometabolic health. Obesity. 2015;23(9):1800-10.

[4] Larsen RN, Kingwell BA, Sethi P, Cerin E, Owen N, Dunstan DW. Breaking up prolonged sitting reduces resting blood pressure in overweight/obese adults. Nutr Metab Cardiovasc Dis [Internet]. 2014;24(9):976-82. Available from: http://dx.doi.org/10.1016/j.numecd.2014.04.011

[5] Kohl HW, Craig CL, Lambert EV, Inoue S, Alkandari JR, Leetongin G, et al. The pandemic of physical inactivity: Global action for public health. Lancet. 2012;380(9838):294-305.

[6] Morris JN. Yoga Para Gestantes - Aula. Coron Hear Phys Act Work. 1953;1111-20.

[7] Tremblay MS, Aubert S, Barnes JD, Saunders TJ, Carson V, Latimer-Cheung AE, et al. Sedentary Behavior Research Network (SBRN) - Terminology Consensus Project process and outcome. Int J Behav Nutr Phys Act. 2017;14(1):1-17.

[8] Douglas K D, Robert T. Complications of Immobilization and Part 1 : Musculoskeletal and cardiovascular complications. Can Fam Physician. 1993;39(1):1428-37.

[9] Teasell R, Dittmer DK. Complications of immobilization and bed rest. Part 2: Other complications. Can Fam Physician. 1993;39(June):1440-2, 1445.

[10] Dirks ML, Wall BT, Van De Valk B, Holloway TM, Holloway GP, Chabowski A, et al. One week of bed rest leads to substantial muscle atrophy and induces whole-body insulin resistance in the absence of skeletal muscle lipid accumulation. Diabetes. 2016;65(10):2862-75.

[11] Brower RG. Consequences of bed rest. Crit Care Med. 2009;37(SUPPL. 10).

[12] Parry SM, Puthucheary ZA. The impact of extended bed rest on the musculoskeletal system in the critical care environment. Extrem Physiol Med. 2015;4(1):1-8.

[13] Bringard A, Pogliaghi S, Adami A, De Roia G, Lador F, Lucini D, et al. Cardiovascular determinants of maximal oxygen consumption in upright and supine posture at the end of prolonged bed rest in humans. Respir Physiol Neurobiol. 2010;172(1-2):53-62.

[14] Van Dyck D, Cerin E, De Bourdeaudhuij I, Hinckson E, Reis RS, Davey R, et al. International study of objectively measured physical activity and sedentary time with body mass index and obesity: IPEN adult study. Int J Obes. 2015;39(2):199-207.

[15] Owen N, Sugiyama T, Eakin EE, Gardiner PA, Tremblay MS, Sallis JF. Adults' sedentary behavior: Determinants and interventions. Am J Prev Med [Internet]. 2011;41(2):189-96. Available from: http://dx.doi.org/10.1016/j.amepre.2011.05.013

[16] King AC, Powell KE, Kraus WE. The US Physical Activity Guidelines Advisory Committee Report - Introduction. Med Sci Sports Exerc. 2019;51(6):1203-5.

[17] Olanrewaju O, Stockwell S, Stubbs B, Smith L. Sedentary behaviours, cognitive function, and possible mechanisms in older adults: a systematic review. Aging Clin Exp Res [Internet]. 2020;32(6):969-84. Available from: https://doi.org/10.1007/s40520-019-01457-3

[18] Biswas A, Oh PI, Faulkner GE, Bajaj RR, Silver MA, Mitchell MS, et al. Sedentary time and its association with risk for disease incidence, mortality, and hospitalization in adults a systematic review and meta-analysis. Ann Intern Med. 2015;162(2):123-32.

[19] Ku PW, Steptoe A, Liao Y, Hsueh MC, Chen LJ. A cut-off of daily sedentary time and all-cause mortality in adults: A meta-regression analysis involving more than 1 million participants. BMC Med. 2018;16(1):1-9.

[20] Hansen D, Niebauer J, Cornelissen V, Barna O, Neunhäuserer D, Stettler C, et al. Exercise Prescription in Patients with Different Combinations of Cardiovascular Disease Risk Factors: A Consensus Statement from the EXPERT Working Group. Sport Med. 2018;48(8):1781-97.

[21] Bull FC, Al-Ansari SS, Biddle S, Borodulin K, Buman MP, Cardon G, et al. World Health Organization 2020 guidelines on physical activity and sedentary behaviour. Br J Sports Med. 2020;54(24):1451-62.

[22] Ekelund U, Steene-johannessen J, Brown WJ, Fagerland MW. Ekelund , U ., Steene-Johannessen , J ., Brown , W . J ., Fagerland , M . W ., Owen , N ., Powell , K . E ., Bauman , A ., Lee , I . (2016). Does physical activity attenuate, or even eliminate , the detrimental association of sitting time with mortalit. Lancet. 2016;6736:972-7.

[23] Ekelund U, Brown WJ, Steene-Johannessen J, Fagerland MW, Owen N, Powell KE, et al. Do the associations of sedentary behaviour with cardiovascular disease mortality and cancer mortality differ by physical activity level? A systematic review and harmonised meta-analysis of data from 850 060 participants. Br J Sports Med. 2019;53(14):886-94.

[24] Dempsey PC, Biddle SJH, Buman MP, Chastin S, Ekelund U, Friedenreich CM, et al. New global guidelines on sedentary behaviour and health for adults: broadening the behavioural targets. Int J Behav Nutr Phys Act. 2020;17(1):1-12.

[25] Chau JY, Grunseit A, Midthjell K, Holmen J, Holmen TL, Bauman AE, et al. Sedentary behaviour and risk of mortality from all-causes and cardiometabolic diseases in adults: Evidence from the HUNT3 population cohort. Br J Sports Med. 2015;49(11):737-42.

[26] Dempsey PC, Larsen RN, Sethi P, Sacre JW, Straznicky NE, Cohen ND, et al. Benefits for Type 2 Diabetes of Interrupting Prolonged Sitting With Brief Bouts of Light Walking or Simple Resistance Activities. Diabetes Care. 2016;39(6):964-72.

[27] Duvivier BMFM, Schaper NC, Hesselink MKC, van Kan L, Stienen N, Winkens B, et al. Breaking sitting with light activities vs structured exercise: a randomised crossover study demonstrating benefits for glycaemic control and insulin sensitivity in type 2 diabetes. Diabetologia. 2017;60(3):490-8.

[28] Healy GN, Dunstan DW, Salmon J, Cerin E, Shaw J, Zimmet P, et al. Beneficial associations with metabolic risk. Diabetes Care. 2008;31(4):661-6.

[29] Thosar SS, Bielko SL, Mather KJ, Johnston JD, Wallace JP. Effect of prolonged sitting and breaks in sitting time on endothelial function. Med Sci Sports Exerc. 2015;47(4):843-9.

[30] Wheeler MJ, Green DJ, Cerin E, Ellis KA, Heinonen I, Lewis J, et al. Combined effects of continuous exercise and intermittent active interruptions to prolonged sitting on postprandial glucose, insulin, and triglycerides in adults with obesity: a randomized crossover trial. Int J Behav Nutr Phys Act. 2020;17(1):1-11.

[31] Climie RE, Wheeler MJ, Grace M, Lambert EA, Cohen N, Owen N, et al. Simple intermittent resistance activity mitigates the detrimental effect of prolonged unbroken sitting on arterial function in overweight and obese adults. J Appl Physiol. 2018;125(6):1787-94.

[32] Saunders TJ, Atkinson HF, Burr J, MacEwen B, Skeaff CM, Peddie MC. The Acute Metabolic and Vascular Impact of Interrupting Prolonged Sitting: A Systematic Review and Meta-Analysis. Sport Med [Internet]. 2018;48(10): 2347-66. Available from: https://doi.org/10.1007/s40279-018-0963-8

[33] Loh R, Stamatakis E, Folkerts D, Allgrove JE, Moir HJ. Effects of Interrupting Prolonged Sitting with Physical Activity Breaks on Blood Glucose, Insulin and Triacylglycerol Measures: A Systematic Review and Meta-analysis [Internet]. Vol. 50, Sports Medicine. Springer International Publishing; 2020. 295-330 p. Available from: https://doi.org/10.1007/s40279-019-01183-w

[34] Bergouignan A, Latouche C, Heywood S, Grace MS, Reddy-Luthmoodoo M, Natoli AK, et al. Frequent interruptions of sedentary time modulates contraction- and insulin-stimulated glucose uptake pathways in muscle: Ancillary analysis from randomized clinical trials. Sci Rep [Internet]. 2016;6(July):1-13. Available from: http://dx.doi.org/10.1038/srep32044

[35] Homer AR, Fenemor SP, Perry TL, Rehrer NJ, Cameron CM, Skeaff CM, et al. Regular activity breaks combined with physical activity improve postprandial plasma triglyceride, nonesterified fatty acid, and insulin responses in healthy, normal weight adults: A randomized crossover trial [Internet]. Vol. 11, Journal of Clinical Lipidology. National Lipid Association; 2017. 1268-1279.e1 p. Available from: http://dx.doi.org/10.1016/j.jacl.2017.06.007

[36] World Health Organization (WHO). No Title. Ottawa Chart Heal Promot [Internet]. 1986; Available from: http://www.who.int/healthpromotion/conferences/previous/ottawa/en/

[37] (WHO) WHO. Preventing noncommunicable diseases in the workplace through diet and physical activity : WHO/World Economic Forum report of a joint. World Heal Organ / World Econ Forum 2008 [Internet]. 2008;Global Str. Available from: https://www.who.int/dietphysicalactivity/workplace/en/

[38] World Health Organization & Burton J. World Health Organization. WHO Heal Work Framew Model Backgr Support Lit Pract [Internet]. 2010; Available from: https://apps.who.int/iris/handle/10665/113144

[39] WHO. More Active People for a Healthier World. J Policy Model. 2018;28(6):615-27.

[40] Shrestha N, Kukkonen-Harjula KT, Verbeek JH, Ijaz S, Hermans V, Pedisic Z. Workplace interventions for reducing sitting at work. Cochrane Database Syst Rev. 2018;2018(6).

[41] Cheval B, Tipura E, Burra N, Frossard J, Chanal J, Orsholits D,

et al. Avoiding sedentary behaviors requires more cortical resources than avoiding physical activity: An EEG study. Neuropsychologia [Internet]. 2018;119(May):68-80. Available from: https://doi.org/10.1016/j.neuropsychologia.2018.07.029

[42] Hagura N, Haggard P, Diedrichsen J. Perceptual decisions are biased by the cost to act. Elife. 2017;6:1-20.

[43] Brand R, Cheval B. Theories to explain exercise motivation and physical inactivity: Ways of expanding our current theoretical perspective. Front Psychol. 2019;10(MAY):1-4.

[44] Hagger MS, Weed M. DEBATE: Do interventions based on behavioral theory work in the real world? Int J Behav Nutr Phys Act. 2019;16(1):1-10.

[45] Zink J, Belcher BR, Imm K, Leventhal AM. The relationship between screen-based sedentary behaviors and symptoms of depression and anxiety in youth: A systematic review of moderating variables. BMC Public Health. 2020;20(1).

[46] Suggate SP, Martzog P. Screen-time influences children's mental imagery performance. Dev Sci. 2020;23(6):1-13.

[47] Wan MW, Fitch-Bunce C, Heron K, Lester E. Infant screen media usage and social-emotional functioning. Infant Behav Dev [Internet]. 2021;62(November 2020):101509. Available from: https://doi.org/10.1016/j.infbeh.2020.101509

[48] Granic I, Lobel A, Engels RCME. The benefits of playing video games. Am Psychol. 2014;69(1):66-78.

[49] Leigh M. Vanderloo PSCPMAMsKTCPJMMCSBMMs. Vanderloo2020. J Dev Behav Pediatr. 2020;41(5):19-20.

[50] Nguyen P, Le LKD, Nguyen D, Gao L, Dunstan DW, Moodie M. The effectiveness of sedentary behaviour interventions on sitting time and screen time in children and adults: An umbrella review of systematic reviews. Int J Behav Nutr Phys Act. 2020;17(1):1-11.

[51] Biddle SJH, Petrolini I, Pearson N. Interventions designed to reduce sedentary behaviours in young people: A review of reviews. Br J Sports Med. 2014;48(3):182-6.

[52] Emara AK, Ng MK, Cruickshank JA, Kampert MW, Piuzzi NS, Schaffer JL, et al. Gamer's Health Guide: Optimizing Performance, Recognizing Hazards, and Promoting Wellness in Esports. Curr Sports Med Rep. 2020;19(12):537-45.

[53] Stojan R, Voelcker-Rehage C. A Systematic Review on the Cognitive Benefits and Neurophysiological Correlates of Exergaming in Healthy Older Adults. J Clin Med. 2019;8(5):734.

[54] Claus GM, Redkva PE, Brisola GMP, Malta ES, de Poli R de AB, Miyagi WE, et al. atric Exercise Science. The article appears here in its accepted, peer-reviewed form, as it was provided by the submitting author. It has not been copyedited, proofread, or formatted by the publisher. 2017;

[55] Warburton DER, Bredin SSD. Health benefits of physical activity: A systematic review of current systematic reviews. Curr Opin Cardiol. 2017;32(5):541-56.

[56] Tremblay MS, Carson V, Chaput JP, Connor Gorber S, Dinh T, Duggan M, et al. Canadian 24-hour movement guidelines for children and youth: An integration of physical activity, sedentary behaviour, and sleep. Appl Physiol Nutr Metab. 2016;41(6):S311-27.

[57] Song C, Gong W, Ding C, Yuan F, Zhang Y, Feng G, et al. Physical activity and sedentary behavior among Chinese children aged 6-17 years: A cross-sectional analysis of 2010-2012 China

National Nutrition and health survey. BMC Public Health. 2019;19(1):1-8.

[58] Königstein K, Klenk C, Appenzeller-Herzog C, Hinrichs T, Schmidt-Trucksäss A. Impact of sedentary behavior on large artery structure and function in children and adolescents: a systematic review. Eur J Pediatr. 2020;179(1):17-27.

[59] Hidding LM, Altenburg TM, van Ekris E, Chinapaw MJM. Why do children engage in sedentary behavior? Child- and parent-perceived determinants. Int J Environ Res Public Health. 2017;14(7).

[60] Rodriguez-Ayllon M, Cadenas-Sánchez C, Estévez-López F, Muñoz NE, Mora-Gonzalez J, Migueles JH, et al. Role of Physical Activity and Sedentary Behavior in the Mental Health of Preschoolers, Children and Adolescents: A Systematic Review and Meta-Analysis. Sport Med [Internet]. 2019;49(9):1383-410. Available from: https://doi.org/10.1007/s40279-019-01099-5

[61] Kehler DS, Theou O. The impact of physical activity and sedentary behaviors on frailty levels. Mech Ageing Dev [Internet]. 2019;180(November 2018):29-41. Available from: https://doi.org/10.1016/j.mad.2019.03.004

[62] Kikuchi H, Inoue S, Amagasa S, Fukushima N, Machida M, Murayama H, et al. Associations of older adults' physical activity and bout-specific sedentary time with frailty status: Compositional analyses from the NEIGE study [Internet]. Vol. 143, Experimental Gerontology. 2021. 111149 p. Available from: https://doi.org/10.1016/j.exger.2020.111149

[63] Brookfield K, Thompson CW, Scott I. The uncommon impact of common environmental details on walking in older adults. Int J Environ Res Public Health. 2017;14(2).

Chapter 6

Lifestyle Transition towards Sedentary Behavior among Children and Youth in Sub-Saharan Africa: A Narrative Review

Lucy-Joy Wachira

Abstract

Worldwide lifestyles are changing with the fastest transition being witnessed in lower-income countries, especially in developing countries like Sub-Saharan Africa (SSA). An influx of easily acquired labor saving screen-based gadgets in many homes has affected many lives. This phenomenon is widespread affecting urban and rural affluent households with income deprived communities playing quick 'catch up' in the belief that this is a sign of prestige. This has led to prolonged sitting hours and excessive screen-based sedentary time especially among children. The high crime rate in urban settings has forced more parents to keep children indoors and "keep them busy" with screen gadgets. Children and youths are vulnerable and easily influenced and habits formed in childhood are seen to be carried forward into adulthood. This chapter highlights the increased sedentary lifestyle of the unique SSA population, whose unique cultural and socioeconomic factors gave them very active lifestyles previously. The plight of children and youth as vulnerable groups; and the resulting effects of sedentary screen-based activities have been discussed. Ongoing monitoring and surveillance of sedentary behavior and time among children and youth in SSA for policy development and strategic intervention is strongly advised.

Keywords: sedentary behavior, screen time, sedentary screen-based devices, physical activity, children and youth, Sub-Saharan Africa

1. Introduction

In addition to meeting physical activity (PA) recommendations, globally, increasing evidence supporting sedentary behavior as a distinct health concern is attracting more attention of public health agencies [1]. Sedentary behavior is characterized by sedentary screen-based behaviors such as television (TV) viewing, computer and cell phone use and video games; and sedentary non-screen-based behaviors involving extended sitting, as in school or in a car [2]. Technological advancements towards automated and less labor intensive performance, even in our daily chores, have led to increased time spent in sedentary behavior. Incidentally, such perceived advancement in lifestyle and labor-saving activities is thought to indicate better living conditions. Unfortunately, instead there is an increase in the incidence and prevalence of chronic-degenerative diseases directly related to low levels of physical activity and excessive time spent in sedentary behaviors. This has now become an urgent public health concern leading to numerous initiatives for raising awareness about risks associated with excessive time spent in sedentary behaviors. Children and youth are the most vulnerable and easily influenced. Despite the perception that children are `naturally' active [3], evidence suggests that they spend a significant amount of time in sedentary activities; and many do not accumulate recommended levels of PA for health [4, 5]. Habits formed in childhood are also carried forward into adulthood [6]. Longer periods of exposure of such behaviors allows NCDs time to develop and severely affect subsequent health [7], thus making it imperative that the foundation for lifelong PA and reduced sedentary time be laid as early in life as possible.

This chapter highlights the physical activity transition and resulting sedentary lifestyle of the SSA population, whose cultural, socioeconomic activities and unique characteristics was previously endowed by a very active lifestyle compared to the rest of the world. Though sedentary behavior has generated tremendous research interest over the past decade around the world, there has be a paucity of data in scientific literature concerning lifestyle habit changes from sub-saharan countries. Perhaps this is because of the attention placed on poverty-associated malnourishment at the expense of a very serious emerging lifestyle change associated with reduced activity.

This chapter will however, attempt to consolodate the findings of the available few studies from SSA to paint a picture of the phenominon. It gives a general understanding of the status of sedentary behavior in various contexts, in the severely under-reported lives of children and youth. The chapter's attention is on the plight of children and youth and their notable increased engagement in screen-based sedentary activities. They require urgent intervention and public health strategies to avert a serious health crisis.

2. The physical activity transition in LMICs in Africa

Worldwide, lifestyles are changing as a result of economic, educational, cultural and technological developments, with the fastest transition witnessed in lower-income countries. One consequence of this, as evident in many developing countries, such as in SSA, is the physical activity transition which is characterized by a change in lifestyle towards decreased engagement in energy demanding activities and transportation activity and increases in less active leisure-time physical activity. While many factors may have caused the increase in physical inactivity and sedentary behavior, cultural shifts, globalization and urbanization, that often accompany drastic changes in lifestyle, may account for this phenomenon in low and middle-income countries [8, 9].

In his explanation of the physical activity transition, Popkin [10] relates the effect of industrialization and modernization to a shift in the energy expenditure patterns and time allocation in most occupations. He also describes the shift in physical effort at home and leisure activities, allowing engagement in increasingly sedentary work.

In Africa, home electrification as well as motorization of farming activities, have transformed daily home chores and time-consuming, often back-breaking, fulltime occupation for the peasant or the working woman. This has also touched the lives of children, even in their education pursuits. In the past, especially in the African rural settings, education activities and programmes took place in outdoors, focusing on nature based learning, survival and experiential learning, characterized by physical engagement and active transportation. We are now witnessing rapid digitization of education materials with an overdependence on screen-based sedentary activities. Most African children, especially in urban settings, now depend on school bus transportation to and from school, perhaps due to dangerous, chaotic heavy traffic and increased crime brought about by modernization.

Possibly, an even more astounding shift has come in leisure time activities. In the past, children were mainly in the outdoors engaging in active physical activities that 'produced a good sweat'. The rapid shift in television viewership, internet connectivity and cable linkages to very many households and many public spaces, as well as motorization of movement and entertainment resorts are now key elements to the shift in leisure pursuits especially in Africa. In the past, leisure activities for children often meant active play outdoors for long hours until it was too dark to play anymore. Unfortunately, today this is characterized by sedentary activity involving screen-based gadgets especially in urban settings [9, 11]. Developing countries, have witnessed an influx of cheap easily acquired and accessible labor saving gadgets that have flooded homes and the lives of children. This is common among urban households and the rural community is quickly 'catching up', perceiving this to be a sign of affluence and prestige. As evident in the few studies, this has led to prolonged sitting hours and excessive sedentary time especially, among children.

Shifts in the physical environment have drastically affected lifestyle in SSA, particularly in high density towns and cities that have been linked to environmental factors ranging from street connectivity, availability of walking spaces, street safety and the organization, layout of buildings and communities. With increased economic advancements, modernization and development, the rural communities are gradually catching on [12, 13]. In an attempt to address this notion, Popkin, [10] advocates increasing opportunities for physical activity, such as public and private recreation facilities, parks, recreation centers and, green spaces. Also recommended are provision for active transportation options, such as sidewalks, cycle paths, high road connectivity, and lower automobile transportation density that will all increase physical activity levels. Further, there is need for legislation to control constraints of physical activity such as crime and air pollution. The neighborhoods in many urban settings in SSA have high crime rates; thus, forcing parents to keep their children indoors and providing screen gadgets to keep them occupied instead of being engaged in active physical activity outdoors.

3. Sedentary behavior

3.1 Physical inactivity and sedentary behavior

Sedentary behavior is distinct from physical inactivity. Sedentary behavior is defined as any waking behavior characterized by low energy expenditure ($\leq$1.5 metabolic equivalents) while in a sitting, reclining or lying posture [14]. Physical inactivity on the other hand describes low involvement in light, moderate, or vigorous physical activity. These two terms are often mistakenly used interchangeably yet there is a clear difference. Being 'physically inactive' means not doing enough physical activity and consequently not meeting the physical activity guidelines while being 'sedentary' means sitting or lying down for long periods. It is possible for a person to have sufficient physical activity and meet the recommended daily PA guidelines, yet still be considered sedentary if they spend a large portion of their day sitting or lying down [15, 16].

Sedentary behaviors are a set of behaviors, with unique environmental determinants and a range of health consequences. There are many different forms of sedentary behavior, especially in the lives of children and youth that include educational activities such as homework, passive traveling such as motorized transport, seated hobbies like reading and talking with friends, and screen time behavior like TV viewing and video games. Although screen time serves as a valuable index for sedentary lifestyle, it accounts for only about a third of total sedentary time [17], with the rest of sedentary time being spent in other sedentary activities [18]. Guidelines that recommend limiting time spent in sedentary behavior [19, 20], focus primarily on limiting screen time and breaking up prolonged sitting. However, there is need for clearer guidance regarding other forms of sedentary behavior, which may also be important for health.

3.2 Sedentary behavior among children and youth

The last decades have seen worldwide notable decrease in PA among young people with concomitant increase in sedentary time, probably due to the drastic increased exposure to screen-based behavior [21]. There is evidence that risk behaviors acquired during childhood may continue into adulthood [6]. Sedentary behavior guidelines recommend that children aged 5 to 11 years should not engage in more than 2 hours of recreational screen time daily as part of a healthy lifestyle. It further recommends that children should reduce motorized transport, long periods of sedentary sitting and time spent indoors throughout the day in order to gain health benefits [22, 23]. Reviewed literature concerning sedentary time found that children spent 6 hours on average in sedentary pursuits during and out of school [24]. The adolescence period encourages independent lifestyle behaviors where they can make independent choices and change behaviors that can have immediate and long-term health impact [25]. Unfortunately, adolescents are found to be the most sedentary of pediatric populations. Evidence shows that they spend 57% of after-school period in sedentary activity [26]. It is also noted that the highest increases in sedentary behaviors may occur during the early adolescence 9 to 12 years [27]. This reemphasizes the notion and risk of sedentary behavior in childhood persisting into adulthood [28]. Therefore, investigation that addresses sedentary behavior and health during adolescence will enhance their present health, improve health over their life course, and protect the future generation's health and wellbeing [29]. There is worrying evidence of increasing levels of sedentariness among school-going children, majority of who do not meet the recommendations for PA, in the developing world [30]. Regrettably, in-depth research regarding sedentary behavior during childhood and adolescence remains poorly described, especially in SSA.

3.3 Sedentary behavior and health and wellbeing

Physical inactivity and sedentary behavior are recognized as important modifiable behavioral health risk factors associated with the development of various chronic diseases and mortality [31, 32]. The WHO classifies physical inactivity as the fourth leading cause of global mortality and one of the greatest health challenges [33]. Physical inactivity and SB are the main causes for approximately 30% of ischemic heart disease cases, 27% of diabetes cases, 21–25% of breast and colon cancers [33] and have also been associated with many other NCDs [34, 35].

Several studies have documented adverse negative effects of increased sedentary behavior on children's health [14, 36–40] and independent of level of PA [41]. Studies have reported associations between higher levels of sedentary behavior and numerous negative health markers that include physical, behavioral and psychological outcomes among the youth [42]. In-depth examination of sedentary behavior during leisure-time is crucial because it has been more consistently associated with health outcomes [39, 43]. Increased sedentary behavior is related to higher depressive symptoms, unfavorable body composition, cardiovascular risk factors, poor physical fitness, lower self-esteem, and lower quality of life [39, 43, 44]. Although evidence varies with specific type of sedentary behavior, there is a link between sedentary behavior and impaired anthropometric, cardio-metabolic fitness and social-health indicators in youth [39, 43]. Studies focused on screen-based behaviors have also found a significant relationship between self-reported TV-viewing/screen time and cardiovascular health outcomes in youth population [39, 43, 45].

3.4 Correlates of sedentary behavior

There is considerable public health interest in understanding the correlates and implications of sedentary behavior on all segments of the population. There are however, unique considerations and challenges when studying correlates of sedentary behavior among children and youth [46]. Current evidence suggests that sedentary time increases with age [47–49] and further investigation of sedentary behaviors across age groups could reveal specific aspects during youth that may benefit future age-targeted interventions. Also noted is lower overall level of actual physical activity in physical education classes, lower levels of PA among adolescent girls than adolescent boys, and decreasing PA levels among girls after puberty [50]. Whereas sedentariness is also inversely associated with socioeconomic status in high income-countries, it is associated positively in low- and middle-income countries with association tending to vary by sedentary behavior domains [51].

In summary, the following have been identified as being positively associated with sedentary behavior during adolescence; among the older age groups, [52, 53], female [53, 54] higher socioeconomic position and income [52, 53, 55], higher parental education and professional level [52, 54], overweight [52], and alcohol use [52]. However, living in the country side [52], being physically active [52–54], parents physical activity level [54], parental and friends supportive of physical activity [54], and having positive perceptions of the neighborhood [54] were found to be negatively associated with sedentary behavior.

Since young people spend considerable proportion of their time at home [56], the physical environment of the house could also exert an important influence on their lifestyle behavior. Factors such as neighborhood design, traffic, and accessibility to green areas or sports facilities are important, bearing in mind the environmental differences and unique characteristics, especially in SSA. For instance, crime and violence in the neighborhood that is linked with urbanization tend to also limit activities outside of the home, limiting outdoor play and physical movement thus increasing sedentary activities among children and youth [57]. Further, higher access to media equipment at home has been related to increase in screen-based sedentary behavior [58]. The influx of screen-based sedentary gadgets, technological advancements and use of labor-saving modern amenities by young people can promote sedentary activities. Given that non-screen based sedentary behavior may represent a high percentage of sedentary time in young people [59], its existing associations and impacts have not been conclusively determined. Further investigation, especially in SSA, is necessary to establish key indicators for purposes of designing targeted intervention and policy.

3.5 Screen-based sedentary behavior among children and youth

One important sedentary lifestyle exploratory dimension among children is determining their time spent engaged in screen-based activities such as watching television, playing video games and computer work [49], collectively referred to as screen time (ST) [60]. As screen-based sedentary behavior is taking over the lives of children and adolescents, it is becoming a key public health concern in managing their health and wellbeing. The influx of electronic media and child focused programming has dramatically increased screen-based sedentary activity. As documented in developing countries, the introduction of video, computer, tablet and internet games, concomitant with saturation of cell phones with built-in games, is rapidly replacing the time that children would have otherwise spent in more physically active pursuits [61]. Seemingly, as screen time increases significantly, physical activity continues to decline. For a long time, the time spent watching TV has been treated as a representative measure of screen time [62–64]. However, TV time alone is not an adequate representative measure of screen time. Many other devices like computers, tablets, mobile phones, and games consoles have now become a common part of the youth lifestyle [65]. Therefore, a more inclusive investigation is necessary when assessing sedentary behavior as a whole, and particularly screen-time among youth. Research reports a significant increase not only in TV time; but in other types of screen time as well. All of which appears to be the driving trend in recent years [66]. Such behavior, especially watching TV, has also been linked to unhealthy eating habits. In fact, researchers have linked unhealthy eating practices to the biological effects of prolonged sitting watching TV and reduced physical activity or a combination of these factors to overweightness and obesity among youth [24].

Given the amount of screen time and screen-based sedentary behavior related to educational activities, there is urgent need for public health guidelines regarding education-related sedentary behaviors both, at home and at school. This is important for teachers and students and policy development. Increasing investigation into the effects of sedentary behavior on academic performance has revealed negative association between [67]. However, it is important to note that the time spent in screen-based activities might be only a small part of the total sedentary behavior of youth during their leisure-time [68], and that each sedentary activity could influence on a youth's academic performance differently. For instance, screen-based sedentary activities related to studying and completing academic homework may be associated with higher academic performance, but entertainment such as watching or listening to music may influence academic performance negatively [69].

In view to the negative impact of screen-based sedentary behavior on the health of young people, Barnett et al. [70] recommend interventions that would reduce television and recreational screen-based time. Strategies could include removal of such devices from the bedroom and where meals are eaten. They argue that this could promote social interaction during meal times and more outdoor activities that do not involve screen devices.

4. Sedentary behavior among children and youth in SSA

Majority of the few studies that have examined sedentary behavior in SSA have non-representative samples that majorly target isolated population groups scattered throughout the region and present inconclusive data. They also do not focus on all aspect of sedentary behavior. In single country studies, there are notable differences in the prevalence and status of sedentary behavior among children and youth, perhaps due to obvious study methodological differences and unique social cultural and geographical characteristics across the continent. There are notable inconsistent findings on sedentary behaviors presenting varying results on sex (boys vs. girls), type of school attended (private vs. public), SES groups (high vs. low), day (weekdays vs. weekend days) and area of residence (urban vs. rural), making it difficult to adequately draw conclusions. There are also a number of multicounty studies on sedentary behavior of school-aged children in sub-Saharan Africa. For instance, a systematic review [9] examined 17 studies and concluded that the reported means of time spent in sedentary pursuits ranged from 1.3 hours to 6 hours on weekdays, and were as high as 8 hours on weekends. The study concluded that the noted urbanization trend suggests an increase in sedentary behaviors over time as the data revealed higher sedentary activity among urban and higher SES children than rural and lower SES children. The following is a summary of research findings from studies in SSA (**Table 1**).

Lead author (reference)	Countries	Age (years)	Main findings with respect to sedentary behavior and physical inactivity
Peltzer [71]	Uganda, Namibia, Kenya, and Zimbabwe	13–15	29.7% in Uganda, 25.7% in Namibia, 43.4% in Kenya, and 43.7% in Zimbabwe reported less than 3 hours of sitting per day.
Peltzer [72]	Ghana and Uganda	13–15	27% of children spent more than 3 hours per day in sedentary pursuits.
Peltzer [73]	Botswana, Kenya, Namibia, Senegal, Swaziland, Uganda, Zambia, and Zimbabwe	13–15	39.4% spent less than one hour per day sitting, and an additional 32.7% spent 1–2 hours per day sitting when not in school or doing homework. Zambian and Senegalese children were the least active (9.0% and 10.9%, respectively).
Malete [74]	Botswana	14	Participants spent an average of 6.2 hours per day sitting. Public school students and those living in rural villages (lower SES) reported significantly more minutes of sitting than students in private schools or those from cities (higher SES).
Omuemu [75]	Nigeria	6–19	35% to 90.7% engage in screen time activities daily. Television viewing and video games were the most common screen-based sedentary behavior, while reading magazines and books for pleasure (45%), followed by listening to music (38%) were the reported non screen-based sedentary behavior. Above 95% of 11- to 19-year-old children and youth in a city of a South–south region of Nigeria spent an average of 3 hours and 15 minutes on the non-screen-based sedentary behavior.
Manyanga [76]	Zimbabwe	5–17	Approximately 75% of Zimbabwean children and youth spend the recommended ≤2 hours per day in sedentary behaviors. About 15% reported watching 5 or more hours of television the previous day. Electronic video games (23%) and watching television (26%) were the most common sedentary behaviors reported among Zimbabwean children and youth.
Benefice [77, 78]	Senegal	13.3 ± 0.5	Participants reported only 1.33 to 1.41 hrs of sedentary time per day. Senegalese adolescent spent 50% of their time in sedentary activities, and most school girls were less active than those who did not attend school.
Garnier [79]	Senegal	13–15	Senegalese girls spent more time in sedentary behaviors than boys (4.23 h *vs*. 2.49 h).

Lead author (reference)	Countries	Age (years)	Main findings with respect to sedentary behavior and physical inactivity
Diouf [80]	Senegal	8–11	Participants spent 65% of their time in sedentary pursuits. All the children presented light PA level and spent most of their time (min/day) in sedentary behavior.
Prista [81]	Mozambique	5–17	Noted substantial increase in sedentary habits due to the growth and availability of the internet in the lives of children and adolescents. There was also a shift from familiar agricultural practices to small trading (involving a lot of sitting), including children traders, which has subsequently led to an increase in their sedentary time.
Ghana Health Services [82] Nyawornota [83]	Ghana	15–19	Between 20% and 70% of children and youth were sedentary. Children attending private schools are more sedentary and more likely to be transported to school in a car, use a computer more often, and watch television not only more frequently but for longer hours.
Ocansey [84]	Ghana	5–17	Over 60% of Ghanaian children do not meet minimum levels of PA for health enhancing benefits. Less than 30% of basic school pupils were transported in an automobile to school every day.
Asare [85]	Ghana	13–18	Ghanaian adolescents perceive walking to school an indication of poverty. 54.1% were highly sedentary with more females being in highly sedentary category than males (52.5% versus 47.5% respectively). Computer and internet use were higher during weekend days than weekdays and made the larger contribution to the total sedentary time of both boys and girls (weekday: 4.65 h/d, 4.08 h/d; weekend: 7.09 h/d, 6.41 h/d). Boys and girls used the computer for similar hours (4.65 h/d, 7.09 h/d versus 4.08 h/d, 6.41 h/d respectively). Private school scored higher on sedentary behavior than those in public school [9.91 (6.37) h/day versus 4.78 (5.71) h/day respectively] mainly because these students in private schools are from affluent homes, and have more access to screen devices, especially the internet and computer games at home.
KNBS [86]	Kenya	15–19	61% of adolescent girls and 36% of the adolescent boys (years) do not engage in continuous physical activity optimally.
Muthuri [87]	Kenya	9–11	Direct measurement of sedentary time among Kenyan children was 398 minutes (6.6 hours), while self-report data showed that urban children spent an average of 1.75 hours in screen-based sedentary activities during the school day and 4.25 hours during weekend days.
Onywera [88]	Kenya	9–12	Higher SES and urban living children in Kenya were found to spend significantly more time in sedentary pursuits than their lower SES and rural counterparts, with approximately 50% of the urban children, and only 30% of the rural children reporting over 2 hours each week on screen time activities.
Ojiambo [89]	Kenya	13 ± 1	Urban children in Eldoret Kenya spent 72% of their wake time sedentary.

Lead author (reference)	Countries	Age (years)	Main findings with respect to sedentary behavior and physical inactivity
Wachira [90]	Kenya	9–11	Overall, children accumulate a lot more recreational ST during weekend days than on school days. Among those that had moderate to-high levels of ST, 75.9% had a TV in their bedroom, 13.8% had a computer, 25.3% had a hand-held video game device, 33.3% had a cell phone, and 19.5% had a non-hand held video game system such as Play-station or Xbox. 76.7% of those who engage in TV viewing over the weekend recorded higher levels of ST. There was a significant association between the overall ST levels and sex ($\chi 2 = 12.036$, $p = 0.002$) and school type ($\chi 2 = 8.340$, $p = 0.015$) but no association with SES. Male participants were 2.1 times more likely to have higher ST levels than female participants (OR = 2.1; 95% CI: 1.32 ± 3.37; $p = 0.002$). Private school participants were found to be 1.5 times more likely to have high ST than public school participants.
Uys [91]	South Africa	10–17	Children seem to not meet the recommended guidelines of 2 hours of screen time or less per day and their social media and cell phone activities recording high usage. Children watched an average of nearly 3 hours of television per day. South Africans are heavy users of social media, averaging 2.7 hours per day, active social media accounts grew by 20% in 2014 and a further 10% in 2015, and youth-dominated Instagram use grew by 133% from 2014 to 2015. These have significantly increased screen-based sedentary behavior.
Micklesfield [92]	South Africa	9	Weekend television viewing among children and youth is higher during weekends, with older children generally presenting higher viewing times.
Lennox [93]	South Africa	15	Children in higher SES schools spent more time watching television than children in lower SES schools on both weekdays and weekends.
Micklesfield [94, 95]	South Africa	11–12 and 14–15	Rural lower socioeconomic status was associated with less sedentary time and more walking for transport. Higher maternal, household, and community level SES were significantly associated with increased sedentary time.

Abbreviations: *KNBS-Kenya National Bureau of Statistics, OR- Odds Ratio, SES- Socioeconomic Status, ST- Screen Time, TV- Television, χ- Chi Square analysis result.*

Table 1.
Summary of research finding on sedentary behavior and physical inactivity among children and youth in SSA.

There is evidence of sedentary behavior among children and youth in SSA but with inconsistent findings across populations. More studies revealed a higher level of sedentary behavior among girls, children attending private school, those from urban areas, and those from high SES than their counterparts. The weekend days seem to attract increased sedentary activity and sedentary time than weekdays. Time is ripe for targeted interventions that focus on such groups while future studies pursue conclusive positions on prevalence and trends in sedentary behavior among children and youth in SSA.

5. Conclusion

This chapter describes the characteristics of the noted transition towards a more sedentary lifestyle, particularly in the lives of children and youth. It also presents a narrative of the status of sedentary behavior among the children and youth in SSA based on published findings of available literature. To the best of my knowledge, there are no existing guidelines for sedentary behavior for children and youth in SSA. Researchers, practitioners and policy developers rely on guidelines and recommendations developed elsewhere [17, 18]. Over the last decade, though sedentary behavior has been a research topic of interest globally, few studies have examined this phenomenon in SSA. The available studies present inconsistent findings that might be attributable to environmental variability, unique social-cultural characteristics across the continent and study methodological differences. They also present inconclusive data focused on isolated population groups scattered throughout the region, making it difficult to present a clear prevalence and pattern of sedentary behavior among children and youth in SSA. Although a large portion of the African population (especially in the rural settings) may not exhibit high physical inactivity, the rapid increase and trend towards higher sedentary time and behavior is now an urgent public health concern affecting population health, productivity and the economy. It is recommended that sedentary behavior, especially among children and youth (a vulnerable group that represent the future workforce), be given priority in research, public health initiatives and policy development.

Author details

Lucy-Joy Wachira
Department of Physical Education, Exercise and Sport Science, School of Public Health and Applied Human Sciences, Kenyatta University, Nairobi, Kenya

*Address all correspondence to: wachira.lucy@ku.ac.ke

References

[1] Active Healthy Kids Canada. Active Healthy Kids Canada. Don't let this be the most physical activity our kids get after school. The Active Healthy Kids Canada 2011 Report Card on Physical Activity for Children and Youth, Active Healthy Kids Canada, Toronto. 2011. dvqdas 9jty7g6. cloudfront.net/reportcard2011/ahkcreportcard20110429final.pdf.

[2] Barnes J, Behrens TK, Benden ME, Biddle S, Bond D, Brassard P, et al. Letter to the Editor: Standardized use of the terms" sedentary" and" sedentary behaviours". Applied Physiology Nutrition and Metabolism-Physiologie Appliquee Nutrition Et Metabolisme (2012): 37(3):540±2.

[3] Livingstone, M. B. E., et al. "How active are we? Levels of routine physical activity in children and adults." Proceedings of the Nutrition Society 62.3 (2003): 681-701.

[4] Guthold, Regina, et al. "Global trends in insufficient physical activity among adolescents: a pooled analysis of 298 population-based surveys with 1· 6 million participants." The Lancet Child & Adolescent Health 4.1 (2020): 23-35.

[5] Marques, Adilson, et al. "Prevalence of Physical Activity among Adolescents from 105 Low, Middle, and High-Income Countries." *International Journal of Environmental Research and Public Health* 17.9 (2020): 3145.

[6] Telama, R. "Tracking of physical activity from childhood to adulthood: a review. Obes Facts 2: 187-195." (2009).

[7] Baird, Janis, et al. "Developmental origins of health and disease: a lifecourse approach to the prevention of non-communicable diseases." *Healthcare*. Vol. 5. No. 1. Multidisciplinary Digital Publishing Institute, 2017.

[8] Hancock, Christine, Lise Kingo, and Olivier Raynaud. "The private sector, international development and NCDs." Globalization and Health 7.1 (2011): 23.

[9] Muthuri, Stella K., et al. "Temporal trends and correlates of physical activity, sedentary behaviour, and physical fitness among school-aged children in Sub-Saharan Africa: a systematic review." International Journal of Environmental Research and Public Health 11.3 (2014): 3327-3359.

[10] Popkin, Barry M. "The nutrition transition: an overview of world patterns of change." *Nutrition Reviews* 62.suppl_2 (2004): S140-S143.

[11] Katzmarzyk, Peter T., and Caitlin Mason. "The physical activity transition." Journal of Physical Activity and Health 6.3 (2009): 269-280.

[12] Cobbinah, Patrick Brandful, Michael Odei Erdiaw-Kwasie, and Paul Amoateng. "Africa's urbanisation: Implications for sustainable development." Cities 47 (2015): 62-72.

[13] Popkin, Barry M., and Penny Gordon-Larsen. "The nutrition transition: worldwide obesity dynamics and their determinants." International Journal of Obesity 28.3 (2004): S2-S9.

[14] Tremblay, Mark S., et al. "Sedentary behavior research network (SBRN)–terminology consensus project process and outcome." *International Journal of Behavioral Nutrition and Physical Activity* 14.1 (2017): 75.

[15] Department of Health, Australian Government. Sedentary Behavior. Commonwealth of Australia 2019. https://www1.health.gov.au/internet/main/publishing.nsf/Content/sbehaviour

[16] González, Karimé, Jorge Fuentes, and José Luis Márquez. "Physical

inactivity, sedentary behavior and chronic diseases." *Korean Journal of* Family Medicine 38.3 (2017): 111.

[17] Biddle, Stuart JH, Trish Gorely, and Simon J. Marshall. "Is television viewing a suitable marker of sedentary behavior in young people?." Annals of Behavioral Medicine 38.2 (2009): 147-153.

[18] LeBlanc, Allana G., et al. "Correlates of total sedentary time and screen time in 9-11 year-old children around the world: The International Study of Childhood Obesity, Lifestyle and the Environment." *PloS One* 10.6 (2015): e0129622.

[19] Canadian Society for Exercise Physiology. Canadian 24-hour movement guidelines for children and youth: An integration of physical activity, sedentary behaviour, and sleep. CSEP 2016.

[20] Physical Activity Guidelines Advisory Committee. Physical Activity Guidelines Advisory Committee. (2018). 2018 physical activity guidelines advisory committee scientific report. U.S. Department of Health and Human Services. 2018

[21] Guthold, Regina, et al. "Worldwide trends in insufficient physical activity from 2001 to 2016: a pooled analysis of 358 population-based surveys with 1· 9 million participants." The Lancet Global Health 6.10 (2018): e1077-e1086.

[22] American Academy of Pediatrics. Policy statement on children, adolescents, and television. *Pediatrics*. 2001 107(2), 423±6. PMID: 11158483

[23] Canadian Society for Exercise Physiology. Canadian sedentary behavior guidelines for children 5±11years. 2011. www.csep.ca/ guidelines.

[24] Lou, D. "Sedentary behaviors and youth: Current trends and the impact on health." *San Diego, CA: Active Living Research* 10 (2014).

[25] Eaton, D. K., Kann, L., Kinchen, S., Shanklin, S., Flint, K. H., Hawkins, J., ... Wechsler, HYouth risk behavior surveillance - United States, 2011. *MMWR Surveill Summ,* (2012). *61*(4), 1-162.

[26] Arundell, Lauren, et al. "A systematic review of the prevalence of sedentary behavior during the after-school period among children aged 5-18 years." International Journal of Behavioral Nutrition and Physical Activity 13.1 (2016): 1-9.

[27] Janssen, Xanne, et al. "Development of sedentary behavior across childhood and adolescence: longitudinal analysis of the Gateshead Millennium Study." *International Journal of Behavioral Nutrition and Physical Activity* 13.1 (2016): 88.

[28] Biddle, Stuart JH, et al. "Tracking of sedentary behaviours of young people: a systematic review." Preventive Medicine 51.5 (2010): 345-351.

[29] Patton, George C., et al. "Our future: a Lancet commission on adolescent health and wellbeing." The Lancet 387.10036 (2016): 2423-2478.

[30] Guthold, Regina, et al. "Physical activity and sedentary behavior among schoolchildren: a 34-country comparison." The Journal of Pediatrics 157.1 (2010): 43-49.

[31] Sheikholeslami, Sara, Arash Ghanbarian, and Fereidoun Azizi. "The impact of physical activity on non-communicable diseases: Findings from 20 years of the Tehran Lipid and Glucose Study." International Journal of Endocrinology and Metabolism 16.4 Suppl (2018).

[32] Lee, I-Min, et al. "Effect of physical inactivity on major non-communicable

diseases worldwide: an analysis of burden of disease and life expectancy." The Lancet 380.9838 (2012): 219-229.

[33] World Health Organization. Global health risks: mortality and burden of disease attributable to selected major risks. Geneva: World Health Organization; 2009.

[34] Prentice-Dunn, Hannah, and Steven Prentice-Dunn. "Physical activity, sedentary behavior, and childhood obesity: a review of cross-sectional studies." Psychology, Health & Medicine 17.3 (2012): 255-273.

[35] Leung, May May, et al. "Intervening to reduce sedentary behaviors and childhood obesity among school-age youth: a systematic review of randomized trials." *Journal of Obesity* (2012).

[36] Marshall, Simon J., and Ernesto Ramirez. "Reducing sedentary behavior: a new paradigm in physical activity promotion." American Journal of Lifestyle Medicine 5.6 (2011): 518-530.

[37] Saunders, Travis J., Jean-Philippe Chaput, and Mark S. Tremblay. "Sedentary behaviour as an emerging risk factor for cardiometabolic diseases in children and youth." Canadian Journal of Diabetes 38.1 (2014): 53-61.

[38] Biswas, Aviroop, et al. "Sedentary time and its association with risk for disease incidence, mortality, and hospitalization in adults: a systematic review and meta-analysis." Annals of Internal Medicine 162.2 (2015): 123-132.

[39] Carson, Valerie, et al. "Systematic review of sedentary behaviour and health indicators in school-aged children and youth: an update." *Applied Physiology, Nutrition, and Metabolism* 41.6 (2016): S240-S265.

[40] Hoare, Erin, et al. "The associations between sedentary behaviour and mental health among adolescents: a systematic review." *International Journal of Behavioral Nutrition and Physical Activity* 13.1 (2016): 108.

[41] Tremblay, Mark Stephen, et al. "Physiological and health implications of a sedentary lifestyle." *Applied Physiology, Nutrition and Metabolism* 35.6 (2010): 725-740.

[42] Felez-Nobrega, Mireia, et al. "Temporal trends in leisure-time sedentary behavior among adolescents aged 12-15 years from 26 countries in Asia, Africa, and the Americas." International Journal of Behavioral Nutrition and Physical Activity 17.1 (2020): 1-11.

[43] van Ekris, Evi, et al. "An evidence-update on the prospective relationship between childhood sedentary behaviour and biomedical health indicators: a systematic review and meta-analysis." Obesity Reviews 17.9 (2016): 833-849.

[44] Gopinath, Bamini, et al. "Physical activity and sedentary behaviors and health-related quality of life in adolescents." Pediatrics 130.1 (2012): e167-e174.

[45] Biddle, Stuart JH, Enrique García Bengoechea, and Glen Wiesner. "Sedentary behaviour and adiposity in youth: a systematic review of reviews and analysis of causality." *International Journal of Behavioral Nutrition and Physical Activity* 14.1 (2017): 43.

[46] Welk, G. J., & Kim, Y. Sedentary behavior in youth. In W. Zhu & N. Owen (Eds.), Sedentary behavior and health: Concepts, assessment & intervention, p221-400. Champaign, IL: Human Kinetics, 2016.

[47] Janssen, Xanne, et al. "Development of sedentary behavior across childhood and adolescence: longitudinal analysis of the Gateshead Millennium Study." *International Journal of Behavioral*

Nutrition and Physical Activity 13.1 (2016): 88.

[48] Ruiz, Jonatan R., et al. "Objectively measured physical activity and sedentary time in European adolescents: the HELENA study." American Journal of Epidemiology 174.2 (2011): 173-184.

[49] Santos, Diana A., et al. "Patterns of accelerometer-derived sedentary time across the lifespan." Journal of Sports Sciences 36.24 (2018): 2809-2817.

[50] Knuth, Alan G., and Pedro C. Hallal. "Temporal trends in physical activity: a systematic review." Journal of Physical Activity and Health 6.5 (2009): 548-559.

[51] Mielke, Brown, Nunes, Silva, & Hallal, 2017 Mielke, G. I., Brown, W. J., Nunes, B. P., Silva, I. C., & Hallal, P. C. Socioeconomic correlates of sedentary behavior in adolescents: Systematic review and meta-analysis. *Sports Medicine,* (2017)*47*(1), 61-75.

[52] Dias, P. J. P., Domingos, I. P., Ferreira, M. G., Muraro, A. P., Sichieri, R., & Goncalves-Silva, R. M. V. Prevalence and factors associated with sedentary behavior in adolescents. Revista de Saude Publica, (2014) *48*(2), 266-274. https://doi.org/10.1590/s0034-8910.2014048004635.

[53] Ferreira, Rodrigo Wiltgen, et al. "Prevalence of sedentary behavior and its correlates among primary and secondary school students." *Revista Paulista de Pediatria (English Edition)* 34.1 (2016): 56-63.

[54] Aznar, S., et al. "Psychosocial and environmental correlates of sedentary behaviors in spanish children." BioMed Research International (2017).

[55] Mielke, G. I., Brown, W. J., Ekelund, U., Brage, S., Goncalves, H., Wehrmeister, F. C., ...Hallal, P. C.. Socioeconomic position and sedentary behavior in Brazilian adolescents: A life-course approach. *Preventive Medicine,* (2018)*107*, 29-35.

[56] Sener, Ipek N., et al. "An analysis of children's leisure activity engagement: examining the day of week, location, physical activity level, and fixity dimensions." Transportation 35.5 (2008): 673-696.

[57] Parajara, Magda do Carmo, et al. "Are neighborhood characteristics associated with sedentary behavior in adolescents? A systematic review." International Journal of Environmental Health Research 30.4 (2020): 388-408.

[58] Tandon, Pooja S., et al. "Home environment relationships with children's physical activity, sedentary time, and screen time by socioeconomic status." *International Journal of Behavioral Nutrition and Physical Activity* 9.1 (2012): 88.

[59] Olds, Tim S., et al. "Descriptive epidemiology of screen and non-screen sedentary time in adolescents: a cross sectional study." *International Journal of Behavioral Nutrition and Physical Activity* 7.1 (2010): 92.

[60] Lanningham-Foster, Lorraine, et al. "Energy expenditure of sedentary screen time compared with active screen time for children." Pediatrics 118.6 (2006): e1831-e1835.

[61] Must, Aviva, and D. J. Tybor. "Physical activity and sedentary behavior: a review of longitudinal studies of weight and adiposity in youth." International Journal of Obesity 29.2 (2005): S84-S96.

[62] Eisenmann, J. C., et al. "Combined influence of physical activity and television viewing on the risk of overweight in US youth." International Journal of Obesity 32.4 (2008): 613-618.

[63] Steffen, Lyn M., et al. "Overweight in children and adolescents associated

with TV viewing and parental weight: Project HeartBeat!." American Journal of Preventive Medicine 37.1 (2009): S50-S55.

[64] Zhang, Gang, et al. "Television watching and risk of childhood obesity: a meta-analysis." The European Journal of Public Health 26.1 (2016): 13-18.

[65] Office of Communications. "Children and parents: Media use and attitudes report 2017." (2017).

[66] Rideout, Victoria J., Ulla G. Foehr, and Donald F. Roberts. "Generation M 2: Media in the Lives of 8-to 18-Year-Olds." *Henry J. Kaiser Family Foundation* (2010).

[67] Tremblay, Mark S., et al. "Systematic review of sedentary behaviour and health indicators in school-aged children and youth." *International Journal of Behavioral Nutrition and Physical Activity* 8.1 (2011): 98.

[68] Biddle, Stuart JH, et al. "The prevalence of sedentary behavior and physical activity in leisure time: a study of Scottish adolescents using ecological momentary assessment." Preventive Medicine 48.2 (2009): 151-155.

[69] Sharif, Iman, and James D. Sargent. "Association between television, movie, and video game exposure and school performance." Pediatrics 118.4 (2006): e1061-e1070.

[70] Barnett, Tracie A., et al. "Sedentary behaviors in today's youth: approaches to the prevention and management of childhood obesity: a scientific statement from the American Heart Association." Circulation 138.11 (2018): e142-e159.

[71] Peltzer, Karl. "Health behavior and protective factors among school children in four African countries." International Journal of Behavioral Medicine 16.2 (2009): 172-180.

[72] Peltzer, Karl, and Supa Pengpid. "Overweight and obesity and associated factors among school-aged adolescents in Ghana and Uganda." International Journal of Environmental Research and Public Health 8.10 (2011): 3859-3870.

[73] Peltzer, Karl. "Leisure time physical activity and sedentary behavior and substance use among in-school adolescents in eight African countries." International Journal of Behavioral Medicine 17.4 (2010): 271-278.

[74] Malete, L.; Motlhoiwa, K.; Shaibu, S.; Wrotniak, B.H.; Maruapula, S.D.; Jackson, J.; Compher, C.W. Body image dissatisfaction is increased in male and overweight/obese adolescents in Botswana. Journal of Obesity *(2013)*: doi:10.1155/2013/763624.

[75] Omuemu, V. O., and C. E. Omuemu. "The prevalence of overweight and its risk factors among adolescents in an urban city in Edo State." *Nigerian Journal of Clinical Practice* 13.2 (2010).

[76] Manyanga, Taru, et al. "Results from Zimbabwe's 2016 report card on physical activity for children and youth." Journal of Physical Activity and Health 13.s2 (2016): S337-S342.

[77] Benefice et al 2004 Benefice, E.; Garnier, D.; Ndiaye, G. Nutritional status, growth and sleep habits among Senegalese adolescent girls. *European Journal of Clinical Nutrition. (*2004): *58*, 292-301.

[78] Bénéfice et al. 2001 Bénéfice, E.; Garnier, D.; Ndiaye, G. Assessment of physical activity among rural Senegalese adolescent girls: Influence of age, sexual maturation, and body composition. Journal of Adolescents Health (2001): 28, 319-327.

[79] Garnier & Benefice 2006 Garnier, D.; Benefice, E. Reliable method to estimate characteristics of sleep and physical inactivity in free-living

conditions using accelerometry. Annals of Epidemiology (2006): *16*, 364-369.

[80] Diouf, Adama, et al. "Physical activity level and sedentary behaviors among public school children in dakar (senegal) measured by paq-c and accelerometer: Preliminary results." *International Journal of Environmental Research and Public Health* 13.10 (2016): 998.

[81] Prista, António, et al. "Results from the Mozambique 2016 report card on physical activity for children and adolescents." Journal of Physical Activity and Health 13.s2 (2016): S213-S217.

[82] Ghana Health Services (GHS). United Nations Children's Fund (UNICEF), Centers for Disease Control and prevention (CDC). Ghana School-based Health Survey. Accra, Ghana 2012.

[83] Nyawornota V. K, Aryeetey R, Bosomprah S, Aikins M. An exploratory study of physical activity and over-weight in two senior high schools in the Accra Metropolis. Ghana Medical Journal (2013): 47(4):197-203.

[84] Ocansey, Reginald, et al. Results from Ghana's 2016 Report Card on Physical Activity for Children and Youth. *Journal of Physical Activity and Health,* 2016, 13 (Suppl 2), S165 -S168 http://dx.doi.org/10.1123/jpah.2016-0272

[85] Asare, Mavis, and Samuel A. Danquah. "The relationship between physical activity, sedentary behaviour and mental health in Ghanaian adolescents." Child and Adolescent Psychiatry and Mental Health 9.1 (2015): 11.

[86] Kenya National Bureau of Statistics (KNBS), ICF International. *Kenya Demographic and Health Survey, Key Indicators*. Rockville, MD: ICF International (2014).

[87] Muthuri SK, Wachira LJ, Onywera VO, Tremblay MS. Correlates of objectively measured overweight/obesity and physical activity in Kenyan school children: results from ISCOLE-Kenya. BMC Public Health. 2014;14:436. PubMed doi:10.1186/1471-2458-14-436

[88] Onywera, V.O.; Adamo, K.B.; Sheel, A.W.; Waudo, J.N.; Boit, M.K.; Tremblay, M. Emerging Evidence of the Physical Activity Transition in Kenya. Journal of Physical Activity and Health (2012): *9*, 554-562.

[89] Ojiambo, R.M.; Easton, C.; Casajus, J.A.; Konstabel, K.; Reilly, J.J.; Pitsiladis, Y. Effect of urbanization on objectively measured physical activity levels, sedentary time, and indices of adiposity in Kenyan adolescents. Journal of Physical Activity and Health (2012): *9*, 115-123.

[90] Wachira, Lucy-Joy M., et al. "Screen-based sedentary behaviour and adiposity among school children: Results from International Study of Childhood Obesity, Lifestyle and the Environment (ISCOLE)-Kenya." *Plos One* 13.6 (2018): e0199790.

[91] Uys, Monika, et al. "Results from South Africa's 2016 report card on physical activity for children and youth." Journal of Physical Activity and Health 13.s2 (2016): S265-S273.

[92] Micklesfield, L.K.; Levitt, N.S.; Carstens, M.T.; Dhansay, M.A.; Norris, S.A.; Lambert, E.V. Early life and current determinants of bone in South African children of mixed ancestral origin. Annals of Human Biology (2007): *34*, 647-655.

[93] Lennox, A.; Pienaar, A.E.; Wilders, C. Physical fitness and the physical activity status of 15-year-old

adolescents in a semi-urban community. South African Journal for Research in Sport, Physical Education and Recreation (2008): *30*, 59-73.

[94] Micklesfield LK, Pedro TM, Kahn K, Kinsman J, Pettifor JM, Tollman S, et al. Physical activity and sedentary behavior among adolescents in rural South Africa: levels, patterns and correlates. BMC Public Health (2014): 14: 40.

[95] Micklesfield, L.; Pedro, T.; Twine, R.; Kinsman, J.; Pettifor, J.; Tollman, S.; Kahn, K.; Norris, S. Physical Activity Patterns and Determinants in Rural South African Adolescents. In Proceedings of the Be Active 2012 Conference, Sydney, Australia, 26-28 September 2012; p. S251.